CLOSE
TO WHERE
THE
HEART
GIVES
OUT

CLOSE
TO WHERE
THE
HEART
GIVES
OUT

A Year in the Life
of an Orkney Doctor

MALCOLM ALEXANDER

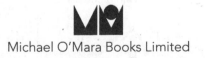

Michael O'Mara Books Limited

This paperback edition first published in 2020

First published in Great Britain in 2019 by
Michael O'Mara Books Limited
9 Lion Yard
Tremadoc Road
London SW4 7NQ

A CIP catalogue record for this book is available from
the British Library.

Papers used by Michael O'Mara Books Limited are natural, recyclable
products made from wood grown in sustainable forests. The
manufacturing processes conform to the environmental regulations of
the country of origin.

ISBN: 978-1-78929-236-7 in paperback print format
ISBN: 978-1-78929-124-7 in ebook format

The title of this book was inspired by the poem, 'Orkney: This Life' in *Into
You* by Andrew Greig, published by Bloodaxe, 2001.

Some names and identifying details have been changed to
protect the privacy of individuals.

Cover design: Natasha Le Coultre
Typeset by Ed Pickford

Printed and bound in Great Britain by CPI Books

www.mombooks.com

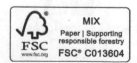

To my eldest son, Martin,
who knows more about writing than I ever will

and

The people of Eday,
who helped me understand the important things in life.

Contents

Prologue

I am who I am and I will be who I will be.

For a young boy to know this before leaving primary school is unusual but this one did: not only did he know what he wanted to be but he knew who. He had seen the man walking down the main street of his village for many years. He had watched his confidence enter the room ahead of him, saw it part the smoke from the coal fire, brush aside the smell of paraffin and ignore the scent of the crisp cleanliness of a newly made bed. This boy carefully observed the nuances of the man's conversation, the details of the examination, his use of percussions, of lookings and listenings with strange instruments. He had marvelled at the strange writing on the pad of paper drawn from the worn leather bag placed at the foot of the bed.

Penicillin V susp 250mg per 5ml
Mitte – 300ml
Sig – 5ml QDS

Visiting the man, he was both fascinated and afraid. Throughout an anaemic childhood he would endure the pain of repeated needle pricks in the lobe of his ear. He was captivated by the dilutions and measuring of his own blood in glass tubes, the smearing and viewing of it under microscopes. This would be followed by further strange writing on the pad of paper drawn from behind the polished leather desk.

Fear and fascination mesmerized him, captivating him, until one day he said, 'I want to be a doctor because I like helping people.'

In time, he would become this man but along the way he would forget why. He would forget the people and try only to solve the puzzles they presented. Hypnotized by the process of illness, by the twists and turns of symptoms, he would forget the effect the manifestations of disease had on real lives. Entranced by medicine, it would take illness and its associated fear to remind him of the reason he wanted to become a doctor all those years ago.

Travelling

I am Eid-ey,
The isthmus isle, the connector of tidal lands.

My birth is deep in the river of time.
My northern rock drawn down from the great
Devonian river
feeding ancient Lake Orcadie.
My southern half compressed from the flooded Lake.
I am hybrid and yet one.
Deposited on the face of the earth and held.

Through time I have travelled.
Leaving the haven of the ancient Lake.
Following the North Star slowly, carefully,
Into the fierce northern seas.

1

Noah's Ark

The little plane cut its engines and descended slowly on to the remote island fifteen miles out in the North Sea. As its wheels touched the rough grass airstrip the pilot opened the throttle once more, roaring the engines into life to control the landing. Rumbling and shaking across the rabbit-burrowed sandy soil of the isthmus that nearly slices the island in two, the plane came to rest alongside the peeling red paint of a wooden shed. An incongruous black and white sign, battered by the wind and rain, said 'London Airport'.

We had arrived on the island of Eday – Eid-ey in Old Norse – the isthmus isle, a place of linking the disconnected. The island was nine miles long and only two miles broad at its widest. Rugged, they said – bleak was a better word. The northern half was brown, covered with brittle wind-blown heather and black peat bog. The southern end was green and treeless, pounded by the sea and scoured by tidal flows. We were there with another young family at the start of a two-day interview for the post of sole general practitioner on the island.

We were watched, carefully observed as the island was presented to us by the interview panel, who highlighted the shop, the eight-pupil school and the surgery. The doctor's house, sitting in a bog of peat with no sight of the sea from any of the salt-coated windows, failed to make it on to the list of notable things.

We said nothing to each other as we sailed back to Kirkwall. The return journey by sea in a chartered passenger boat making sure we had the full experience of island life. In the cabin, still under the eye of the members of the next day's panel, Maggie and I only exchanged glances, smiles with minute unhappy inflections at the corners of our mouths. Her blue-green eyes were dark, and she held her head in a way which made her long, brown pigtail appear rigid, as it transmitted her unhappiness. After eight years of marriage, many of them working together in hospital, we don't need words to communicate with each other. We wouldn't apply for the post. The job was challenging enough as a single-handed doctor on the island twenty-four hours a day. The place was awful, the house and surgery ancient and uncared for by the Health Board. The medical equipment was non-existent. We needed to move away from city-based practice but not that much.

That evening we spoke openly, frankly talking through the reasons for wanting to move. The bickering dissatisfaction of my current practice; their failure to give me a full partnership after four years; the overwhelming sense of sinking into mundane repetitive routine that was nothing like the life either of us had wanted. Deep down I hated what I had become. A technically competent doctor who had lost sight of the people he was treating. Only now and then minor glimpses of the family general practitioner I saw as a child broke through. Maggie would have to give up her part-time work in a neighbouring practice as well, perhaps only occasionally working for me, if that was possible. In the end we decided that I would go to the interview the next morning and allow the panel to decide for us. I would take the job if they offered it – and they did.

August and we were nearly ready to go, leaving Glasgow for Orkney and the island of Eday, which would be our home. Four boys, Martin, Matthew, Michael and Murray, the eldest six years old and the youngest just a year. All preparing for an adventure that none of us really understood. The haunting difference between working with a hospital, ambulances, colleagues all nearby, and working alone on an island with only a tenuous plane link to anywhere in an emergency. The dramatic change from a school of three hundred pupils to one of eight. The challenge of only one shop and supplies that come once a week on the boat. The isolation from all the people we know in our support network. All this we knew but didn't realize how unsettling it would feel until we started to cut the cords holding us to the city.

'Don't prevaricate, boy!' an examiner once said to me. 'Make a decision and move on.' Obviously, this was a surgical exam.

Good advice if you're trying to make a single choice but this move wasn't like that. It was breaking up families and friends, displacing grandparents, aunts and uncles, making adopted grannies redundant. The only thing that wouldn't be broken were ties with colleagues; there were no bonds there to break. It was shifting places. Not from similar to similar but from comfort to ... well, we really didn't know what. Certainly, it will dissolve our safety net of people and make us rely solely on ourselves. The night three months ago in Kirkwall when we talked things through, trying to balance matters before the interview the next day, we were attempting the impossible. You can't balance risk, you just have to take it. Don't prevaricate, boy!

What had seemed to be a perfectly sensible, if slightly eccentric, way of living in suburbia proved quite tricky to transport north. While we thought it was natural to have ducks and geese in our garden in Glasgow, accompanied by a free-range rabbit and a dog, perhaps it wasn't. The actual logistics of animal transfer hadn't featured high on my list of things to do either. Putting the house on the market, telling our friends, extricating myself from the practice, these had all been activities I knew I needed to work through.

Eventually I succeeded in making a ramshackle crate of wire and nails that held our three geese for the journey. Our youngest son, Little Murray, was so excited about travelling 'w'sh a zoo' as he put it. He wasn't so keen after three days of driving with smelly animals. The other animals were not quite so difficult to organize. Spot, our rabbit, travelled with Otto, his guinea pig companion, in their hutch in Maggie's car and the six ducks lived in the boot for the journey. Robbie, our dog, just curled up on the floor as usual. That seemed like a sensible idea. At that moment, anything seemed sensible compared to the lunacy of moving our comfortable suburban zoo to that bleak house.

The time for us to leave arrived and the large blue McAdie & Reeve removal truck pulled up in our street. Weeks of packing disappeared into the back of the huge lorry as slowly the home we had created was dismantled, piece by piece. The polished floor of the large front room re-emerged. Hours, days of work had gone into sanding the beautiful hardwood boards back to their natural colour. I can still see the August sun streaming through the wide bay windows, making the boards gleam. The cherry-wood dining table and chairs vacated our ornate dining room, with its hand-painted cornicing in green and gold. Beds and bunks came down the broad carpeted staircase, the only carpet we had when we moved in. Outside, the gardens slowly filled with a queue of furniture and boxes waiting to be packed in the correct order.

Early next morning the journey began, taking us through landscapes which were familiar at first, until after three days a new window opened on a world we knew almost nothing about. A journey from urban domination to insignificance. Motorways, roads, tracks and ultimately the sea. A city left behind, with its glass and concrete crushed against Victorian sandstone. Redundant shipyards, their skyline claimed by derelict cranes. Urban flyovers which swung past office blocks crammed with workers perched like birds in their glass cages. Contained rows of people looking inwards and ignoring the world outside. Slowly these receded as the sharp edges of the urban cage were blunted by the encroaching greenness of the countryside. I'd never really thought of the countryside as hard before, but the city is no match for it. Viaducts carrying trains and canals stretched higher and higher above the road as we travelled north. As if the land was pushing the urbanization away from itself, holding it at arm's length, rejecting it. Our first day's journey was almost complete when we finally crossed the Moray Firth at Inverness. The road pushed us high into the air as we swept in convoy over the Kessock suspension bridge, completing our sense of leaving and taking us into the Black Isle.

After a full day's drive up the winding A9, we arrived at our destination beside the sea in Rosemarkie and set up camp at the far end of the campsite. Carefully we corralled our car, van and caravan behind a thicket of gorse and whin bushes, secretly letting the geese out of their cage and allowing them to graze a little on the thin machair grass, all the time hoping they didn't start honking and attract the warden. The other animals had to stay in their houses. I doubted we could have caught the ducks if they had decided to head off and the rabbit would have disappeared in an instant.

The next morning, we left the last vestiges of urbanization behind as we continued north. The industrial harbour area of Inverness quickly receded in the rear-view mirror; almost immediately we were surrounded by an alien landscape as we swung over Struie Hill to the Dornoch Firth. The heather that remained in the distance the day before was right beside us on the road as we drove further into the countryside, the road no longer able to force its way through the terrain but instead being forced around it and over it. The long slow climb from Helmsdale started the beginning of real driving as we twisted and turned our way up the mountain edges along the very rim of Scotland. The ultimate test came as we descended again at Berriedale. The hill down was so steep the van screamed in second gear while I stood on the brake as we crept forward; the near hairpin bend at the bottom gave no leeway for mistakes. No sooner had we reached the riverbed than we were off climbing again, mostly in first gear, up through another hairpin bend while the van groaned its way up. A cloud of white smoke and steam belched from the exhaust as we dragged our way up the steep brae.

Suddenly the land changed as we swung inland, cutting across the northern tip of Scotland to reach Thurso. Rock gave way to the vastness of the Flow Country, huge expanses of peat bog reaching back south to the mountains. The only signs of civilization were occasional croft houses, the dwelling houses of the micro-farms scratched from the hillside, the land around them peppered with outhouses and crumbling barns. Old rusting tractors and farm machinery disintegrating in the rain while scraggy sheep clung to the low hills bordering the bog's northern edge. In two days, the transformation was complete. The countryside had taken full charge of all that happened here. Everything shaped by the wind and weather.

We set up camp for the second night, looking down to the harbour at Scrabster and the boat that would take us across the water to Orkney. Even in August it was still much lighter than down south and at ten o'clock at night the islands were clearly visible in the distance. A string of cloud rested along the top of Hoy – like a net curtain along a windowsill.

Our third morning began gently with a sense of peace as we sailed out into the Pentland Firth. A feeling that deepened, cruising along the west coast of Hoy and seeing the patchwork of fields in green and gold perched on the clifftops. A group of low croft houses appeared in a small bay, the name of which I didn't yet know, immediately followed by the giant stack of the Old Man of Hoy dominating the shoreline. There was a permanence about the scene unmatched by anything in the city. The shore slid slowly past as the boat corkscrewed across the waves, rising and falling in the westerly swell. The whole experience was like being on a carousel at a fair, going up and down as pictures surround you, and events not in your control unfold.

Finally, the boat swung easterly into Scapa Flow and the window on our adventure was opened wide. The low rolling hills of mainland Orkney were very similar to those of my childhood in the Borders of Scotland. The little town of Stromness, though, was like nothing I'd seen before. Stone houses tumbling down the steep hillside to crowd the water's edge, some stepping into the waves like rocks jutting into the sea. Little promontories of green were planted with brightly coloured washing on lines and white painted derricks for swinging goods up from rowing boats. The blues and reds of their upturned hulls, drawn up on the shingle beds between jetties, caught in the early morning sun. The windows of the shy homes were all small, reluctant to let you see what went on inside. There was a permanence in this scene too, an unchanging resilience stated simply by 'being'.

2

Into the Sea

It's 5.30 a.m. on Kirkwall pier on the fourth morning of travelling north from Glasgow. My second sea journey is about to begin and I slowly drive our van into position. The wheels bump over the thick white rope net and come to a halt. Gradually, the operator of the little crane raises the net around the sides of the van, making it look like a small whale ready to be lifted into the boat. Then, and without any warning, the whole catch swings into the air. There's a cacophony of honking from the back of the van as our geese take fright. They've been remarkably quiet for most of the journey, but this sudden upward movement seems to be too much for them. The weight of the load in the boot immediately tips the van backwards and it prepares to slide out the net. Then it careers forwards, swinging and dipping like a nodding dog as it spins over the side of the boat and into the hold. My heart is in my mouth when I hear a voice beside me.

'Aye, they lost a Morris Minor last week ch'ust like that.' The voice is thick with an Orcadian accent as he continues, 'You'll be the new doctor for Eday then.'

'That's right, we're heading out today.'

'They nets are tricky things. Still, it made it into the hold,' he says with a twinkle in his eye. 'Take care, Doc.'

He turns and walks away at the very moment a new blue and orange tractor is easily hoisted into the hold, spinning and bouncing over the ship's side before plummeting from sight. A little ripple of amusement goes through the knot of passengers waiting to board.

How does he know who I am? In fact, everyone on the pier seems to know who I am and I've never seen them before. Dad and I board the boat, perhaps ship is a better term for her, as she's very smart in her black and white paint, her narrow bow sitting proudly in the water. Below decks we go to the dining room to search out breakfast. Pushing open the heavy wood and brass door, we are met with the unexpected sight of rows of tables covered with thick white linen cloths. Each cloth is held in place by silver clips, which grasp the raised lips of the table. Places are set with full silver service, the china teacups and plates all corralled by the table edge to prevent them sliding off in stormy seas. Smartly dressed attendants deliver our full cooked breakfast as if we are in a five-star hotel. This is the *Orcadia*, one of the ships that will bring supplies to us on the island, along with her older partner, the cargo boat MV [Merchant Vessel] *Islander*.

'This is quite a ship,' says Dad, who's come north with me to help me set up the house.

'We didn't see this one when we came up for the interview,' I say. 'We came back on the little passenger launch, the *Mariana*. The one Maggie and Mum will come out on tomorrow with the boys.'

'I think we got the better deal; this breakfast is very acceptable. Are you ready for the work today? We've a lot of carpets to lay.'

'No choice, have we? We'll manage, I've had a little practice over the years,' and our conversation drifts on throughout our breakfast.

Sitting at sea level, the waves run just below the portholes and once again the shoreline streams steadily past. Unlike the crossing from Scrabster to Stromness on the snub-nosed MV *St Ola*, this ship cuts into the water, pushing the waves aside. There's no roller coaster like we had alongside the Old Man of Hoy when the long Atlantic waves were reflected back from the cliff face. The rock and seaweed-draped shorelines scroll through the little round windows which frame the scene with salt-encrusted brass circles. It is so much like watching an old wartime movie that at any moment I expect to see a German U-boat surface.

The Green Holms, the rocky islands to the south of Eday, are first to slip over the horizon once we leave the mainland of Orkney and the western shore of Shapinsay behind, then the long beach of Warness appears. Names I've learned from the map now stuffed in the glovebox of the van. Other names become real too, as we round the point into Backaland and tie up at the stone pier that will be our lifeline from now on. We're 250 miles as the crow flies from our home outside Glasgow. Not far by today's standards but after four days of travelling it is becoming clear that this journey isn't solely about distance. There's a feeling of time slipping backwards that first started when we sailed along the coast of Hoy and into Stromness. This has been made more intense by the morning's sail on the old ship and is becoming more detailed still as we land. An old green 1960s Bedford coal lorry is waiting on the pier beside two sea-encrusted Massey Ferguson 135 tractors. Tractors I used to play on as a child. Each vehicle is attended by a stocky man in faded overalls. The oldest of the three stands relaxed, comfortable in an orange boiler suit and flat cloth cap.

Everything we own is now stacked on the pier, ready to be brought up to the house in the truck and tractors that have been waiting for us. Each crate is hoisted and spun out again from the hold of the ship before being bounced once more on to the cobbled surface of the grey-stone pier. Behind us the offloading from the *Orcadia* continues as the pier slowly gathers the week's supply of food and other essentials for the island. Then, with an absence of fuss, she slips the lines holding her fast and resumes her journey to the next of the four islands on her circuit of the North Isles, her hold still crammed with pallets of animal feed, boxes of groceries, more pallets of paint and ironmongery.

Leaving the men on the pier to load our things, I drive the van the four miles north to the house and, once over the final hill, slowly descend to Heatherlea. The house still looks uninspiring as I draw up in front of its wooden garage. The paint on the little blue gate to the yard peels and flakes off as I squeeze through. I reach the crumbling front door and put my shoulder firmly to it, and grudgingly it gives and allows me in. Inside, the dismay at the house returns, the same dismay that nearly stopped us accepting the post at all. Compared to our own beautiful home in Glasgow this place is worse than our memory of it. Empty, cored out and now abandoned after a long period of indifferent Health Board care. Like an old lady putting on make-up to go out for the day, the fresh magnolia paint on the walls only highlights the wrinkles and cracks. The kitchen has been accessorized by our new landlords with newly fitted units and worktops, but the newness only magnifies the dilapidation around us. There are no gleaming wooden floorboards, no ornate cornices, no wide sweeping stairs. All of those and more are left behind. Now there's only a grubby, uncleanable, ancient bathroom, tired rooms and draughty, ill-fitting windows that make the place cold even in August. The electric storage heaters give out a desultory tepid air as they struggle to warm the house. The excitement of the journey north and the sea crossings slips away.

Dad and I stand in the yard, waiting for the first consignment of removal crates to come up from the pier. Now comes the test of the order we packed them in five days ago. I'm not hopeful at all, as my mood swings through cycles of apprehension and depression. First out of the containers should be carpets and my toolbox, along with kitchen essentials. The guttural sound of the old Bedford engine signals the arrival of the first load. As Stan, the local haulier who met us at the pier, draws up we're standing with our fingers crossed outside the decaying front door. Swinging the gate open, he comes in miraculously preceded by a familiar roll of red and grey striped carpet. I've just led Stan upstairs when a woman's voice calls up to us.

'Does anyone need a cup of tea? I thought you might need a hand, is your wife here?'

'Oh hello, I'm Malcolm. Yes, tea would be good, but we haven't got anything sorted out yet.'

'I have,' she says, coming up and joining us. 'This used to be Carol's room when we lived here. She loved that little fireplace – the chimney makes a terrible noise in the winter though. I'm Claire, in case you don't remember, the district nurse.'

'Of course,' I say, relieved that she has reminded me, 'your husband was the GP here twelve years ago, was it? No, Maggie isn't here until tomorrow. My mum is helping her just now with the boys. This is my dad, we're the working party.'

'Right, I'll leave you to it. Tea's in the kitchen when you're ready.'

The rest of the morning is a hectic whirlwind of activity, moving furniture and kitchen equipment. There's a line of tractors outside with goods on the trailers, boxes piled on boxes, all gathered from the pier and rumbled carefully up the four miles of road. Wardrobes that took two men to lift into the truck down south are hoisted easily up the stairwell by Murdo, Claire's son-in-law. No sooner have Dad and I roughly laid one carpet than the room's furniture arrives to hold it in place. At nearly one o'clock I stop to have a break and look out the bedroom window into the walled garden below. A line of six Khaki Campbell ducks toddle through the weeds, heading for the bucket of water we gave them first thing this morning. In another corner of the undergrowth three geese, abreast, are starting to mow the grass down, working slowly in line across the coarse lawn. Maybe we will get things sorted out after all.

Dad and I continue to direct the stream of boxes into each room. Mysteries for the boys to open when they arrive and rediscover the toys lost for over six weeks. It probably seems like a lifetime when you are their age.

The kitchen has slowly sunk under an avalanche of utensils, pots, pans and our supplies of food for the winter. We weren't sure what to expect so the room is now filling slowly with bags of flour, sugar, cereals and crates of tinned food. It looks more as if we are going on an expedition than moving house. Gradually, we push the overabundant supplies into vague order in the cupboards and clear some space to sit down.

In the late afternoon, the tidal flow of people slowly subsides. Dad and I are just sitting down to another cup of tea when there's a quiet but firm knock on the door and a man in his early sixties confidently strides into the kitchen. It's clear immediately that he knows his way around the house as he makes his way towards us, his eye briefly surveying our roughly placed furnishings.

'Good afternoon, I thought I would wait until now to look in,' he says, taking off his tweed cap and sitting down in what you imagine would have been his preferred chair.

'Hello, I'm Malcolm,' I say, stretching out my hand for what seems the hundredth time today.

'You seem to be progressing well. I'm Trevor, the locum GP,' he says, as things become clearer. 'It's pretty hectic moving house, isn't it?'

After introducing my father, we make our way through what will become our dining room and open the connecting door to the surgery, which Trevor is keen to show me. I must admit I haven't even looked in here yet in the rush to prepare the house. Perhaps I should have; it might have prevented the look of dismay on my face as we go in.

The connecting door leads straight into the waiting room. A dismal, dirty, magnolia-coloured corridor with wooden bench seats along both walls and a tiny window at the end. It reminds me of the worst of school cloakrooms. Halfway along the wall a door opens into the yard and opposite this is the entrance to the surgery itself. Pushing open the light, hardboard-covered door, we step into the surgery. The room is completely empty with the exception of the old torn examination couch and a table that doubles as a work desk. The surgery is as desolate as the house.

'I've written out a list of patients who may need to see you soon,' says Trevor, sweeping the pile of dust back from the table edge. 'I didn't use the surgery this week,' he adds unnecessarily.

'Nessie is struggling a bit with her asthma just now but she should be fine,' he continues. 'She's just down the road near the Co-op. Ina has been troubled with her back, you should see her next week, Claire will need to show you how to get there, though. The rest of the list is pretty straightforward.'

I'm not really listening. The room is much worse than I remember now it's devoid of any semblance of a medical environment. The table at which Trevor is still talking is piled with boxes containing the medical files, all of them in the old 5-inch by 7-inch Lloyd George envelopes. There's a computer and keyboard so thick with dust that I would be reluctant to switch it on without a fire extinguisher handy.

'He didn't use the computer much,' Trevor says, again unnecessarily. 'Your colleague preferred to write things down. All the details are on the Lloyd George files.'

I'm still not listening. Walking through into the pharmacy, the shelves are piled with bottles and boxes of pills. There's a thing like a pressure cooker in one corner and a set of thin glass tubes set into a wooden stand that immediately triggers a memory.

'Oh, I see he has a haemoglobinometer,' I say as I have a flashback to my GP's surgery as a boy. Memories of the multiple needle sticks and blood tests of my childhood flood back.

'Dr MacKenzie used to check my anaemia with one of those,' I add as Trevor looks blankly at me.

'I don't think that was his,' he says. 'I imagine Claire will tell you it was her husband's, Dr Bennett, before he died.' He rises to go. 'Okay, if you need me I'll be staying at the north end with the Traills as usual. My phone number is on the paper along with my home address. I'm very happy to come back as your locum when you need me, I've several friends here now.' He turns and opens the surgery door. 'One last thing. I'm leaving on the morning flight, at nine o'clock. So, I'll hand over to you then. I'm sure you'll enjoy it here. Give my regards to your wife when she arrives. Good day!' And with that he leaves.

Standing in the residual debris of the previous doctor's practice, the realization dawns that I have become the doctor, the medical service for this little windswept lump of green and brown hills rising above the wave tops. If anything happens I must deal with it. There is only me. I'm stunned and start to aimlessly push patient record envelopes around in the volcanic amounts of dust that have settled on the table.

I carefully tease one of the buff-coloured envelopes out of the boxes in front of me. The official-looking wallet is quite thick, crammed with similarly coloured individual cards, each recording details of medical treatment over the passing years. The patient details are written in black fountain pen in the requisite boxes on the front.

Surname: Heddle

(with a single line drawn diagonally through it and 'Eunson' neatly added beside it)

Forename: Agnes
Date of birth: 2 October 1919

(just after the First World War and perhaps nine months after Private Heddle returned to his native Orkney)

Each address is recorded in different handwriting as Agnes Heddle moved house. Linkertaing to Millquoy, Millquoy to Toab on mainland Orkney, Toab to Millquoy and finally Millquoy to Number 3 Bu Cottages. A history in place names. Presumably her father moved from Linkertaing ('the Viking meeting place') to Millquoy ('the mill farm'), changing farms to work as a labourer. Then Agnes married and moved to Toab, returning to Millquoy later as her parents grew too old to work the croft, before finally moving to Bu Cottages, where she is now. There's a lot of history on this front page, more than I'm used to seeing on the records in Glasgow, which have been sanitized into large A4 folders to contain all the information needs of modern medicine. Folders which in the process have lost the concise distillation of events held in a Lloyd George envelope.

Easing one of the record cards out, I have something in my hand I haven't seen before. This is a complete medical record of an adult life. Each episode of care is detailed in the language of medicine – hieroglyphs, abbreviations, numerical recordings, all taking up no more than two lines on the card – and is followed by similar lines each winter. A mixture of Greek, Latin and English concisely summing up each encounter.

As I gently squeeze the card back into place in the envelope I finally realize what it is I'm holding. Agnes Eunson – this is Nessie's medical record, spanning her life since the NHS began in 1948. Agnes Heddle – Nessie Eunson – has lived almost all her life on Eday, moving only briefly to mainland Orkney after the First World War. A sense of timelessness is captured in the details recorded on this unassuming buff envelope. A feeling of a chain that remains unbroken. I've never seen a patient's life laid out in one place like this before. A life I'm responsible for now, a whole life stretching day after day, not just an episode of illness needing individual corrective treatment.

Rushing out to the van, I start grabbing the bags of medical equipment and medicines packed in anticipation of the isolation. The realization of just where I am cuts into me. If I don't have everything ready to treat a patient, no one else will do it for me. The Emergency Doctor Service won't take over at night and let me sleep, the ambulance won't arrive and take the patient away. There is only me. Airways, masks, nebulizers, needles, syringes, emergency drugs for every condition I could think of, from post-partum haemorrhage, croup, asthma to heart attacks. The list is endless – or so it seems. What might happen? When might it happen? Will I know what to do? There's nowhere really to lay the various items down so I sweep the dust from the examination couch with my arm, creating a cloud that glitters in the sunlight, making me sneeze.

Gradually, my pile of emergency equipment is set out in a neat row, each item placed in its relevant grouping for ABC. Airway; Breathing; Circulation. Always ABC but now also D and E. I imagine D for damage – trauma, with all its consequences. E is for exposure in my mind – protection against the elements – the wind and rain featuring for the first time in my life when I think about caring for a patient.

After half an hour I begin to slow down. Reassured, perhaps, by the row of familiar things in front of me. Tools I know how to use and some I haven't yet understood. I was offered a set of Kielland's forceps before I left Glasgow, a bizarre-looking arrangement of oddly shaped spoons curving like cupped hands, with a clamp and separator on the handles. They would be used to help a mother struggling to deliver her baby. I have no intention of using these. I'm not even certain which way up they go. I suppose the person who offered them to me may have felt they were coming home since the original design was Norwegian. Perhaps the Vikings influenced the shape. I'll stick to the little set of Wrigley's forceps to help me lift out a reluctant baby. What am I talking about? I hate obstetrics. Two patients intimately entwined, both likely to run into trouble at the same time. If my first emergency is an obstetric one, I'm done for.

Just as I'm descending into panic again, the surgery door opens and Stan pokes his head round.

'Where do you want the last boxes, Doc? They were left on the pier until now.'

'Ah.' I had hoped we were finished with boxes. 'I think we'll just put them in the garage for now, Stan.'

'Aye, fine. You okay, Doc? You look a little pale.'

'I'm fine, Stan, just tired after the travelling.'

'Right you are, I'll get these in the garage then leave you to it. Trevor is away in the morning, isn't he? I'll catch him at the plane when I open the airstrip up. Sleep well.' And he's gone.

Sleep isn't easy and I spend most of the night half-dozing, half-awake as my mind meanders through the past few days, until the alarm clock finally goes off at 8 a.m. Saturday morning and there's only the distant sound of the waves lapping on the shore coming in through the open bedroom window. No sound of aircraft taking off, cars on the street outside, dogs barking in neighbours' gardens; just the sea splashing in the out-of-view bay below us. Weaving through a maze of boxes, I make my way down to the kitchen, the bubbling of the kettle boiling only the second sound of the day. The place is still pretty disorganized, but Dad and I find enough for breakfast and sit in the quiet for a few minutes. The last moment of peace before the boys arrive with Maggie and my mum at ten o'clock.

Our stillness is broken by a knock on the door, and Trevor strides in with the same confidence as the day before, only this time he doesn't sit down.

'Good morning. Sorry to barge in but I'm just off to the plane,' he says. 'Here's the pager should anyone need to get in contact with you. You know to put the phone through to the hospital if you go out, don't you?'

I nod in uncertain agreement.

'The phone numbers are on the list in the surgery; it's pinned to the wall beside the phone. Right, I must be going, or I'll miss the plane. As I said yesterday, let me know if you want me to come back as your locum – I'm pretty free now I've retired. Good luck!' And he leaves, shaking my hand as he goes.

So, this is it. It's me now. Standing bemused in the kitchen, looking blankly at the pager's green light blinking in the palm of my hand. I'm uncertain what I should do next. Nothing, I suppose, but wait.

Settling

I am Eid-ey,
The isthmus isle, the connector of tidal lands.

A place of Settling in troubled seas.
Bridging – Connecting – Linking across time and tide.
Drawing all to me, gathering them on my shores.

The birds will sing my shore songs
and my grasses whisper secrets
Only to those who hear.
My wind and seas shape and form,
Test all who come.

He can rest for now, this settler on.
Before his Testing.

3

The Tilley Lamp

The rest of the weekend disappears in a flurry of excited boys. Boxes are slowly emptied and flattened for return to the removers, furniture moved around, then put back, then moved again until the house begins to look a little like a home. All of a sudden, it's 8.30 a.m. on Monday morning and there's a Land Rover at the front door, waiting to take Martin and Matthew to their new school. At 9 o'clock I turn the key in the surgery door to open it for morning surgery. There's no one there. No cars on the road. No one walking. Going to the yard gate, I look hopefully up the hill to see if there's anyone coming from the south. No one. Just a lazy gull cruising high in the sky.

I don't ever remember sitting in a surgery waiting for patients. In Glasgow we had an open system each morning where anyone could come and sit down to be seen. On a Monday morning there could be thirty patients waiting to see me by 8.30 a.m. A sea of faces looking expectantly at me as I swung open the door to the waiting room, all of them with nothing much wrong. Apart from that one person in the room. The needle in the haystack whose story would be just different enough to make you sit up and listen. Usually, it was just a never-ending stream of coughs, colds, anxiety, backache (both real and convenient). My senior partner had a saying for how to manage this workload.

'Never let their arse hit the seat, son!' he would say and have the prescription written before they sat down. It wasn't so straightforward for me, as I tried to uncover the secret potions he gave the little old ladies.

'Dr Johnstone always gives me a pick-me-up. It comes in a brown bottle,' they would add helpfully.

Unfortunately, the contents of the brown bottle weren't always as clearly recorded in the notes as they might be. Mixtures of syrup of ipecac, pholcodine and even barbiturates in low dose all appeared. Sometimes there was nothing in the mixture except some quinine. To survive, I chose the least noxious substances of no clinical value when I had to give in and provide something. Lots of bitter syrup was dispensed.

In the middle of this flow of nonsense, much of it created by us in the practice continuing to pander to minor symptoms, there would be a real cough. The first signs of a cancer perhaps.

'I only coughed the blood up once, Doctor. I always get an antibiotic at this time of the year but I'm going to stop smoking this time.'

The same words time after time, or is it? This time it's different. Why?

'Have you lost a little weight?'

There's also a look in his face. Slightly haunted, anxious, as if he wants to tell me something but is afraid to do it. Is this the needle in the haystack?

'I think we'll do a chest X-ray just to be sure, shall we?'

Maybe it is something or nothing, but the story is just a little different. The whole story, the words and movements and the looks. I needed to find out.

Today, however, I would be very happy for 'someone's arse to hit the seat'. Half an hour later and still there's no one in the waiting room. I decide to tidy up a bit and start clearing the dust. It's not quite shovelled out into the yard but almost. Arranging the files of notes on the table in what I hope looks like an official manner, I then go in search of the box packed with my other surgery equipment. Once I've positioned a blotter on the desk in front of me and put some pens in place I move the blood pressure machine about until I'm happy with it. Then I move it about some more. I gather the prescription pads into the drawer beside me along with the sick-lines, and sit back. Then I move the blood pressure machine again. I wish someone would just come in and give me something to do.

Sitting back in the comfortable basket chair we've chosen for the surgery, I pretend there's a patient, showing them in and seating them in the other chair. Then I move the chair a little as I can't see them. The computer monitor is the size of a small television and is taking up most of the desk. Sitting where I am, it's directly between me and my patient, blocking them from view. I'm beginning to understand why the previous doctor didn't use it. It's too big. I'll have to start again.

Gradually the hour slips past and eventually the various items on my desk have settled into the right place. For the moment. I haven't dared to switch on the computer yet – it definitely needs to be hoovered out first – but it is now behind me and I can swivel round to use it if I'm feeling brave.

I should tackle the little pharmacy room next. It's only when I go into the large cupboard and start to organize the boxes and bottles into date order that I see the note. Carefully left by my predecessor, it details the administrative tasks needing done. He's also left a little bundle of infectious disease forms with which to notify the Health Board if I need them, which is disconcerting. On the grey laminate worktop there's a tin for collecting the prescription charges and forms to send in each month to the Health Board with a cheque for the amount gathered. Beside this is a note of the name of the local chemist in Kirkwall, from whom I can have my supplies of medications sent out to me. Order on a Monday and collect in person from the weekly boat on a Wednesday. This all seems pretty straightforward, even though I've never had to do any of these things before. Running the practice doesn't bother me. The unexpected emergency is the real anxiety.

After an hour or more of tidying and organizing I need a coffee. Walking through to lock the surgery door, I brush past the examination couch, still carefully set out with all my emergency equipment. The Wrigley's obstetric forceps catch the sunlight. A malevolent little glint bounces from their spoon-shaped handles, which have arranged themselves in a slight smile as they lie there taunting me with their threat of obstetric emergencies. I grab them round the neck and stuff them quickly in a drawer. I've had enough of them panicking me every time I see them.

In the kitchen, I can see that Maggie is also rearranging things the previous person (me) has left. The table is covered with all the tins and dry goods that Dad and I had put away.

'There's mouse droppings everywhere,' she says. 'Didn't you wipe out the cupboards before you stuffed them?'

'Yes, I did. I thought it was just that the place had been empty and they'd wandered into each cupboard.'

'Well, they're clearly still here, and have you done anything about the bathroom? It's impossible to get clean. I had to bath Murray in the sink this morning.'

'I phoned Euan at the Health Board this morning. He wasn't very happy, but he's agreed to put in a new suite. I didn't really give him a choice.'

'Would you like a coffee?'

'I wasn't sure you'd found it yet. Yes please.'

Just as I'm curling my fingers round the steaming mug, the door to the kitchen opens and Claire walks in.

'It's only me, how you getting on? You must be Maggie,' she says as she walks towards her, holding out her hand.

'Would you like a coffee? We've found it now,' Maggie says as she pulls out a chair for Claire.

'Perfect. Strong and black please. How was your first surgery?' she says, turning to me.

'It wasn't,' I say. 'There was no one there. Did I get the time wrong? The list said there's one at 9 a.m. each Monday morning.'

'Ah no, that's all right. The patients will be letting you settle in first. You might get some before the week's out. Trevor told them all to get topped up with medicines last week to give you some time.'

I have difficulty getting my head round this information. I remember the two old ladies with head colds who waited for more than an hour and a half for me while I dealt with a seriously injured man in a car crash. And the father who barged into my surgery because he wanted his perfectly well son seen immediately. Here, people will wait until I'm settled in. Why would they do that? While I think about this Claire continues.

'Someone said you're a doctor too, Maggie. Did you work before coming up here?'

'I worked one day a week, in a practice near Malcolm's and, before that, I was in a partnership in the east end of Glasgow.'

'Brilliant! Will you work here too? The women would love it.'

'I'll need to see how the boys settle in first. Perhaps I could take a surgery once in a while.'

Maggie and Claire continue to chat, while I go through to the surgery to tidy a little more and lock up. I like the idea of Maggie and me working together again, I'll need to see if the Health Board will allow it. Previously, when we worked in hospital, Maggie, then training to be an anaesthetist, used her maiden name professionally. There were some interesting situations when, together, we treated the same patient. Quite often, as the patient wakened from the anaesthetic she had administered, they confided in me, as I completed the plaster designed to hold their fracture in place. They would make statements such as, 'Ah! She's a wee cracker, that doctor,' and, more riskily, 'I wouldn't mind a night out with her.' I took pleasure in delaying my response, pleased that they had noticed how attractive she was but also savouring the moment when I said, 'You've met my wife then.' Maggie had a similar opportunity when she heard a visiting colleague chat me up, after we had all worked together on a patient. The devilment glowed in her eyes as she delivered the killer statement, 'I didn't know you knew my husband so well.' We definitely work well together.

When I come back into the kitchen from the surgery, Maggie and Claire have already made plans to start a mums and toddlers group. It seems they will get on very well, which is great, as I was concerned Maggie might feel isolated in such a small community. As Claire gets up to leave we agree to meet up tomorrow morning to go and see Ina at the south end together. Ina is a little shy, so I should be introduced or she may not say much to me. Once Claire leaves, I decide I have to do some sort of medical work. Sitting around all day just waiting isn't going to help; it's making me anxious. I need to be a doctor to settle my nerves. Picking up the pager from the surgery I write down the paging number and leave it beside the phone in the hall for Maggie. Then, for the first time since we arrived, I walk out to the yard and leave the house behind. As the VW Polo rolls down the hill away from the house and the phone, it feels as if I'm stretching an umbilical cord which will inevitably break. What if something happens when I'm out? Should I really wait at the house in case? Stupid of course, but I feel vulnerable away from the phone. It's not that I haven't done house calls before. In Glasgow, I didn't even have a pager. If I was needed there would be a message at the next patient's home. The difference is there was always someone back at the surgery if a patient turned up unexpectedly needing help. Someone would dial 999 and the ambulance would take the patient away to hospital. Here, the responsibility is all mine now and I'm uneasy.

Having taken the risk of leaving the house, I stop the car half a mile away – half a mile! I could hear Maggie shout to me if she needed me! Number 3 Bu Cottages is a grey harled bungalow in a group of ten homes built by the council. It looks like any other council home I've seen – which is disappointing. I knock on the door and go in with a tentative call of, 'It's the doctor.'

Nessie is sitting in her living room beside her electric fire in a high-backed modern chair. Another disappointment. When I had thought about doing house calls on the island, I pictured peat-burning stoves, black kettles, iron-black pots. I could be anywhere in a Glasgow suburb in this modern little house. Taking more time to look round the room, I see Nessie is surrounded by great cones of wool of all colours. On the table behind her, near the window for the light, there's a strange-looking machine. A grey plastic drum-like cone encircled by needles at the top, with an odd thing like a small crane above it. The table is covered in what looks like woollen jerseys that have been dissected and laid out for forensic inspection. A body split down the side, an arm ripped from wrist to shoulder. On the plastic drum, I see another piece of material impaled on the spikes at the back.

'You'll be the new doctor. Come and sit by the fire.'

'Thank you. I'm Dr Alexander. How are you doing? Dr Grant said you haven't been well,' I say, maintaining the formality I'm used to.

'Ah, Trevor worries too much,' she says, calling Dr Grant easily by his first name. 'I'm fine now, just the asthma catching me out again. He said I should stop working with the wool and I would feel better but how can I do that? I've done it all my life.'

'He's maybe right, though, but I understand. What is it you do with all this wool? It doesn't look like knitting.'

'I'm a linker, I put the garments together that Eileen of "The Bu" farm knits up. I've done it since I was a girl.'

'Even when you were out at Linkertaing?'

'My, how did you know that? That's a long while ago.'

'Ach well, I did a little reading.'

'No, not at Linkertaing, I was too young then. Then it would just be the knitting, simple things like cloths and such.'

Once I've checked her over and adjusted her medication, we chat on for half an hour. There's no rush for me. She'll probably be the only house call today. Nessie has always worked with wool. Initially knitting traditional patterns by hand but then progressing to joining up garments that others knit. She shows me the machine on the table with its wool running through the little crane. The crane bobs up and down, threading the wool through the material captured on the spikes. The edges are flexible when they're finished, stretchy so the knitting doesn't rip when it's worn. A good linker, it seems, is worth their weight in gold and makes good money. A bad linker can ruin days of work with a poor seam.

Just as I'm about to leave she says, 'You'll be ready for the winter then, Doctor?'

'I hope so; the house seems very dependent on electricity, though. I'll need to get a supply of candles and such.'

'Have you not got a Tilley lamp then? They're better than candles and you get a heat from them too.'

'I haven't seen one since I was a boy, Nessie.'

'Right, away and look in the cupboard beside the door and you'll see two of them. Bring the one without a mantle in it.'

Doing as I'm told, she checks it over then hands it to me.

'Right, that's yours now. Ask at the shop and get two spare mantles. You'll see much better with that than candles.'

Despite my protests, she makes me take it and I promise to look in again next week to see how she's doing. Just as I'm closing the door behind me, she calls out once more.

'Mind on and get meths and paraffin too, Doctor.'

And at that single sentence, there I am. Doctor. I feel more comfortable as I drive up to the shop a few hundred yards away. Doctor. I am 'The Doctor'. Slowly, I let the realization settle in and begin to allow myself to wear the title here in this new alien setting.

That evening I put the Tilley lamp together, fitting the gas mantle from the shop. I feel like a child again, watching my father carefully pour methylated spirits into the little brass collar that clips around the long stem leading to the mantle and glass shade. At the base of the lamp there is a tank of paraffin, which you pressurize by pumping the miniature bicycle pump set into the tank. The theory is that the pressurized paraffin jet rises into the long stem where the heat from the collar of meths turns it into gas. Once it's warmed up, the whole thing keeps itself going.

I loved physics and chemistry at school, so I know exactly what I'm doing. The boys have gathered round to watch as I pump up the tank and then light the collar of meths. The blue flickering flame surrounding the stem is the only light in the room, reflecting in four sets of intense eyes. I strike a match and open the valve at the top of the stem to let the gas into the mantle. There's a satisfying hiss as I put the match to it. The hiss is immediately followed by a roar and then four simultaneous screams, as the boys dive under the table and a jet of flame shoots out the top of the lamp, scorching the ceiling.

'What on earth are you doing?' demands Maggie, who has just come back into the kitchen.

'Dad's made a flamethrower, Mum,' says Martin. 'Look, he nearly set fire to the ceiling.'

Tears are rolling down my cheeks as I remember a similar incident with a Primus stove I wasn't supposed to have when I was eight years old. I've always loved setting fire to things.

Before trying again, I let the meths burn for longer to thoroughly heat the stem, then light the mantle, which ignites with a satisfying growl, filling the room with sound and a pleasing white light. I leave the lamp on the table after carefully replacing its glass shade.

Once the boys have gone to bed, I settle peacefully into the armchair in the corner of the kitchen and watch the light flicker around the room. Memories of shadow puppets and ghost stories drift back from my childhood. Unexpectedly, I'm a boy again, peeking round the kitchen door, squinting between the bedsheets hanging like giant creepers from the pulley, suspended over a paraffin stove in an attempt to get them dry. Secretly, I watch our family doctor examine my sister as she lies dazed on the sofa. She'd tripped on three concrete steps in the garden and knocked herself out. She isn't sure where she is, who she is and doesn't remember falling. The doctor's brown leather Gladstone bag lies open beside him while he methodically shines lights from complicated torches into her eyes and ears. He palpates, listens, bends and taps her arms and legs. Lights, tubes, hammers with rubber ends all come and go from the brown leather bag. There's no hesitation in his actions, just the steady rhythmic movement of a man following a long-practised routine. Confidently, he proclaims that my sister will be fine. There's no need to disturb her further with a trip to hospital. Call him if she doesn't wake up properly in two hours. The image is imprinted on my memory next to the thought he would be deemed negligent today, even though he was right. Nowadays, we would do a skull X-ray and consider an overnight hospital stay. I doubt if I'll ever be that confident to take a risk like he did; asserting she didn't have any internal bleeding in her brain based solely on his examination and experience.

The next morning, I find Claire's croft at the south end of the island and together we go to see Ina Flaws. Driving back towards the pier, Claire suddenly asks me to stop and turn on to a grassy track along the side of a field. I would never have noticed it. After a quarter of a mile of driving on a surprisingly smooth cobbled surface, we come to a clutter of uninhabited buildings marooned in fields of cows. I pull up at the side of an old barn. The morning sun picks out the patterns of lichen on the sandstone, stone worn and pitted with years of weathering. Ragwort and milk thistle grow tall around the base of the barn, watered liberally when the rain drips from the rusting corrugated iron roof. There's no sound at all except the quiet ripping of grass as the cows crop their way round the fields to a backdrop of curlews calling on the distant shore. Wind shakes the tall grasses beside the path.

Perhaps Ina is in the barn tending to a calf. Claire signals for me to follow her, and as I round the end of the barn I see another building made of the same stone, sheltering in the barn's lea. This long, low building is roofed with huge flagstones, each grey with lichen but carefully capped at the top with freshly concreted ridging stones. Following the path worn through the long grass, we pass wooden racks set out like the legs of old trestle tables, the aged wood split and cracked by the sun and wind. Each rack is hung with fish, split open lengthways head to tail and hooked like open books over wooden pegs to dry in the sun.

Opening the ill-fitting door set halfway along the building, Claire points out the two bright steel buckets, one at each side of the door. Each bucket is positioned to catch rainwater from the galvanized metal guttering I had failed to notice as we came up to the house.

'There's a well to the back of the house,' says Claire, 'but Ina prefers the rainwater for drinking.'

'Is there no mains water here?'

'No, Ina could have it but she doesn't see the need. She would hate the disruption.'

'How does she bath herself?' I whisper.

My question goes unanswered as we gently intrude upon a century long gone. The doorway is a Narnia-like entrance to a world rarely seen. The kitchen is virtually bare, with the exception of a blackleaded range cooker set into a splendid wall of polished blue and cream tiles. Peats burn silently in the grate and the room is smoky with the scent of burning heather. The only light filters through two tiny windows on the far side of the room, shafting through the thin smoke and picking out the single place setting on the scrubbed wooden table. On the wall opposite the cooker, a blue and white larder cupboard displays various packets and tins in a neat array. A heavy white porcelain sink with no taps hangs beneath one of the windows and completes the kitchen equipment. A single plate, cup and spoon are set out to dry on the wooden draining board. There's no fridge, no washing machine, no appliances of any kind. There's no electricity.

Waving me through into the only other room, Claire calls to Ina to let her know we're here. This room is nearly as bare as the kitchen. Two armchairs, fading with age, sit either side of an open hearth with a peat fire set ready for lighting later in the day. Three old photos hang in their frames on the wall, farming folk and a man in a postman's uniform standing beside a bicycle. A small, thin voice replies from somewhere in the room, but I can't see anyone. Claire parts a pair of heavy brocade curtains covering a recess that shares a wall with the kitchen range and speaks again to a bundle of bedding in the box bed.

A peat-coloured face appears from beneath the layers of covers, shining green eyes looking warily at me.

After careful introductions, Ina lets me examine her. Her increasing back pain has been more troublesome over the past few weeks. Reaching into the recess I try to check her over but find it almost impossible, hanging over the raised edge of the bed. The wooden board enclosing it, worn smooth with years of use, prevents me actually getting near enough to examine her. Eventually, I give up and climb over the shiny wooden threshold into the bed, kneeling in the enclosed sea of blankets. A slight dampness percolates through my trousers from the bedding below. Once I've located Ina and arranged the bedclothes so I can thoroughly check her, I see that not only is her face the colour of peat, but her hands and arms are as well. She is scrupulously clean though, the peat simply ingrained into her skin from years of living and working with the oily brown fuel.

'Ina was born in this bed, Doctor,' says Claire as she supports Ina for me to listen to her chest. 'Her father was the blacksmith here on the farm.'

'I've never stayed anywhere else. When I was young I slept through in the kitchen, next to the range. Now I'm here, since my mother died twenty years ago.' Her voice is soft, almost a whisper.

'Willa comes in as her home help,' adds Claire. 'She'll make her tea later.'

'My uncle was likely the first Orkney soldier killed in the Great War, you know. That's him when he was young, helping my father out with the horses,' she says, pointing to the largest of the three pictures on the wall.

'Ina never married,' says Claire. 'What with the war and then the Spanish flu outbreak, there weren't enough men around, were there!'

'I've never missed them. Always been able to do for myself until now, Doctor. You need to sort out this sore back so I can get up again.'

Clambering back out the recess, I arrange my glass bottles in order on the floor and select a 20ml syringe to take blood samples with. I might as well do as many as I can in the one visit.

'If you're quick, you'll just make the plane,' says Claire, 'It's due in at twelve noon today. Just leave me and I'll walk back home, it's only ten minutes.'

I hadn't even thought about the plane or how I was going to get the samples to the laboratory. I was simply doing what I do down south. Giving Ina some stronger painkillers for now, I'm just about to leave when I spot another Tilley lamp sitting on an oval table beside the window.

'Oh, I've just been given one of these,' I say as I hurry to the door.

'I know,' says Ina. 'Nessie had her father's old one but she'd no use for it,' and she disappears beneath the blankets once more.

How does she know that? I only just got it yesterday and she's never been out of bed. Promising to come back, I dash to the car in a hurry to parcel the blood samples for the plane. In the surgery, the individual tubes are quickly labelled and packed into a little travelling case I found in a cupboard. Then I look up the phone number of the lab and call them to let them know the samples are coming.

'That's fine, Doctor, nice to speak to you,' says Ian from the lab. 'Did you remember to spin the samples for biochemistry before packing them?'

'Spin them?'

'Yes, any plasma samples will need to be spun in the centrifuge before you send them, or the results won't be valid.'

'Ah, right – how do I do that?'

Ian explains that the strange-looking pressure cooker thing I saw the day we arrived is in fact a centrifuge. I need to put my blood sample into the special tubes and spin them fast for ten minutes. This will separate the cells from the plasma and give a better reading. If I don't do this the salts will leak from the blood cells and give me falsely high values.

I carefully empty my sample into a centrifuge tube then fill an identical tube with the same amount of water. This tube is placed directly opposite the blood sample in the little carousel to balance the mechanism. I close the lid and gradually increase the speed to maximum for ten minutes. After the time is up, a simple but fascinating thing has happened. My sample is now in three layers. Liquid on top over a creamy-looking layer and, underneath, the clustered red cells. Using a plastic pipette, I carefully syphon off the liquid and put it into a separate tube for analysis. There's something uniquely satisfying about doing this. As if I'm participating in the analysis, not just collecting samples for others to work on. It seems to bring me closer to my patient too, actually handling Ina's blood, taking care with it and preparing it correctly. I'm feeling pleased with myself when the plane roars overhead. I can just see the tailplane out the pharmacy window as it dips over the hill to the airstrip.

Bundling myself into the car again, I race down to the airstrip with my precious cargo and slide to a halt on the gravel outside the wooden hut.

'No need to rush, Doc. Have you got those blood samples from Ina there then?' asks Stan, now in the role of airport manager and not haulier.

'Erm – yes,' I say, not sure about confidentiality. How did he know I had samples to send?

'Right then, we'll get them away for you. Claire called to say you had some.'

'Did she say who they were from?' I asked, making up my mind to remind Claire about confidentiality.

'No, no, she can't do that. I saw you at Ina's this morning when I was down the pier and you haven't been anywhere else yet today,' he said matter-of-factly. 'I'll pop in later and make sure she has enough peat for the night.'

Confidentiality seems to be an interesting concept on the island. Kind of a two-way street of knowing things that you shouldn't but using them to help out.

Days gather into weeks as we settle on to the island. Routine becomes established, visiting the pier each Wednesday to collect things ordered on the phone from Kirkwall. Rhythm in each day is punctuated by either morning or evening surgeries now regularly attended by the folks on the island. Ina surprised me by readily agreeing to go into Kirkwall to see the surgeon and have her back pain assessed. I thought she would be unwilling to travel but with enough painkiller on board she clambered into the plane and away she went. She would stay with a friend in Kirkwall who she spoke to each week on the phone. I hadn't noticed a phone in her room, but it must be there. Some technology is acceptable then.

Autumn stretches on before us as Maggie and I slowly tidy the little surgery, painting and decorating the whole place until we're happy that it looks comfortable but still clinical. The house is improving too, now we have a new bathroom suite and the old draughty windows have been replaced with modern double-glazed units. The downside of the window replacement is noticed on windy days – which are most days; instead of draughts coming around the window frames they now come up through the floor. The carpet in the living room does an excellent impression of Aladdin's flying carpet. To try to counteract the loss of heat, I've decided to fit a solid fuel stove in the kitchen. Luckily, there's a good chimney in place already and all I need to do is open it up. With help from the local handyman/craftsman/crofter – everyone has at least three jobs – I install a Morsø Squirrel. The little matt-black stove glows quietly on the hearth while carefully drying all our clothes on the pulley swinging above it. If I pack it with coal at night and shut the air intake tightly, it keeps the house warm all through the night. We're ready for the worst of the winter.

Except there doesn't seem to be any winter. The autumn continues into November. In the early evening we drive across the airstrip to Doomy Beach and play in the moonlight. Matthew finds an old fish box stamped 'F. Dibben, Poole, Dorset', with strings of goose barnacles hanging underneath it. Although technically these are barnacles they look like bunches of beautiful blue-grey mussel shells, bound together by long strands of string, holding on to the box in a ropey tangle. Box and barnacles, a drifting island in the sea carried north by wind and tides until it was thrown ashore on this beach. As the moon rises, shimmering the wet sand on the mile-long beach, I wonder if we're a little like the barnacles. Clinging together and pushed north to Doomy Beach.

Another weekend, we see a pod of thirty pilot whales

swimming along the same beach. The grey torpedo shapes cruise along the coastline below us as we walk the West Side Road above the beach. It's not clear if they are lost, confused by the shallow gradient of the sands, or whether they are just checking the island out. Measuring it, plotting its position on their map of the world, making sure it hasn't moved. After three days the visitors are gone into the ocean.

Geese come in waves throughout the autumn and early winter. Flights of barnacle geese land in squadrons on the hill above the airstrip. Their black and white heads and striped blue-grey wings so similar to the markings on the goose barnacles that it was once thought the geese hatched from goose barnacle trees. Perhaps the ones we saw on the beach have just hatched. Greylag geese join the flocks and feed outside our bedroom window, calling nervously to each other through the night. The arrivals and departures seem to follow a rhythm, a respiration with an intake and exhalation of wildlife. Smaller birds arrive in breaths too, finches and buntings appear and disappear in days. Briefly resting on the stunted trees in the garden, then blowing away. None of this activity is sudden or rushed, there is just a natural blush of life that flows around the shorelines and over the hills. The peacefulness is infectious.

Or, at least, it was, until Maggie decided to treat the boys by making sweets – candy-balls to be precise.

Neither Martin nor Mike can have sweets from the local shop, due to their allergies, so home-made sweets have been added to her repertoire. The kitchen fills with the aroma of boiling toffee, while the gang of energetic, peace-shattering helpers gather for the final stages of preparation. A marble slab is laid near the centre of the worktop, ready to receive the hot, caramel-brown liquid. I watch as she pours the near boiling contents of the pot onto the marble while, simultaneously, holding the boys back from the danger. There is no chance of them reaching out too soon – Mum has told them not to. In a similar situation, I would have to repeat the instruction to them several times, before they would understand.

The next and final stage of making the candy-balls is swift. As the liquid begins to set on the slab, Maggie rolls the still hot, pliable toffee with her bare hands, forming it into a long sausage. Then she picks it up and stretches it further, before rolling it again. Each episode of rolling is preceded by a flick of her long pigtail, as she leans forwards. Throughout this process there is still no hint of movement from the waiting boys, who are now armed with pairs of kitchen scissors. At precisely the correct moment, she allows each boy the chance to cut off half an inch of cooling toffee from the long sausage shape. Almost miraculously, small, triangular-shaped sweets fall onto the waiting greaseproof paper. Even Little Murray takes a turn, guided carefully by Maggie.

At the end of the process we have two large jars of candy-balls, four unscathed children, and a husband full of admiration for how his wife achieved the whole thing safely. I hope I never have to take her place, as there could easily be carnage if I try to imitate her.

That evening, just as I'm settling down to read my book on whales and dolphins, a candy-ball firmly wedged in my cheek, the phone rings. My heart jumps when it rings in the evening: I'm still waiting on the impossible emergency. The thought is stupid, I can do this job. There's a long sigh as I wander into the hall to sit at the telephone seat and take notes for the house call. No need, it's Jenny to say would I mind popping in tomorrow to take a look at Tommy, as he has one of his colds coming on. Oh! There was another matter she wanted to discuss with me but that would wait until morning. Placing the phone back on the hook, I'm left with an uneasy feeling that the second item is the more important one on the agenda. Maybe my heart was right to jump.

I've seen Jenny once or twice at the surgery, always with her husband, Tommy, and every Sunday afternoon in the church. The overwhelming impression she gives is of a small bundle of tightly packed energy; her lively pale-blue eyes look at you firmly beneath a large chestnut-coloured wig, its long wavy hair falling to her shoulders. As she gained years – she is now more than seventy – she has lost hair and the story goes that she once spotted this wig at a sale of work and decided that it was the thing for her. Unfortunately, no one has ever shown her how it should be worn, so the whole ensemble sits slightly to one side, pointing in a direction somewhat shy of true or even magnetic north. This gives her head an appearance of being slightly unscrewed at the top. To think, however, that this effect also applied to her character is to commit a grave error, which she would quickly disabuse you of with a single look. When Jenny sets her mind to do something, 'it' is going to happen whether 'it' wants to or not. Even in the short time I've been here I've learned this lesson, and that is what concerns me about the 'other matter' she wants to speak about.

Tommy and Jenny's little house is modern by island standards. Not one of those concrete block and grey harled boxes that Nessie lives in but one of the new breed from the 1950s when prefabrication was the thing after the war. It's a wooden house which they had built beside the traditional flagstone roofed building that was the original family home. Too damp now for continuous habitation, the older building is used for Sunday school and Women's Guild meetings which are held in the sitting room. The house sits just off the road on the hill above the pier, next to the school where Tommy works as caretaker. The easterly views are spectacular over the sound between us and Sanday. The broad seascape spread before you is never still, with the constant wind playing on the water, creating infinity patterns and cats' paws on the surface. Below you, the fields fall gently down into the rippling water until two miles further on they rise softly from the waves, clothed in luxuriant green. Then, folding over the low-lying sandy soil of our neighbouring island, they sink slowly again into the restless North Sea. Not an easy place to concentrate on anything, which is why the school nearby, with its east-facing windows, has high windowsills so the children can't see out. The greenness of the south end of the island contrasts starkly with the brown heather-clad patchwork of the north end. Almost like two different islands taped together by the airstrip in the middle; a hybrid of rocky red sandstone in the north and soft grassy green in the south.

Tommy and Jenny's house itself is minute. Its exterior wooden tongue-and-groove panelling is perfectly painted in cream. The windows are neat, windproofed, with small glass lights that give the house the look of an oversized doll's house. All of this sits below a neat red roof. The entire frontage of the house is made up of a tiny porch to the right of the main Georgian glazed sitting-room window. No need to knock, as Jenny's eagle eye spotted me long ago. I've just enough room to turn around in the tiny porch before Jenny leads me through to the bedroom at the back of the house, squeezing past the little hall table and brushing against a collage of old black and white family photographs on the walls. Family groups standing outside stone steadings, fields with haystacks and horses, all being handworked. A little history of island life on a wall.

I don't think either Tommy or Jenny are more than five feet tall, and the house was obviously built to suit them rather than someone my size. The bedroom is jam-packed with necessities and curios. There are shelves on the wall with china ornaments and more photo frames. The dresser is of a 1950s-style wood-and-glass-topped variety with worn brass handles and is equally crowded with lace doilies, scent bottles and powder-puff jars. There's also one of those wooden shop display stands for hats that's clearly the nightstand for Jenny's wig. The interior reinforces the impression of a doll's house that's been played with for too many years by a child kleptomaniac. I can just see Tommy in the deep multi-blanketed bed and, stepping over two floral chamber pots, I'm able to examine him while Jenny waits for me in the sitting room.

Tommy is fine, but he needs to step up his asthma inhalers for a week or two until the cold settles. I ease myself down into the armchair in the sitting room while Jenny, her wig at a particularly jaunty angle this morning, hands me a cup of tea in a Crown Derby china cup and saucer.

'I wonder, Doctor, what you think about the church?' she says.

'In what way, Jenny?' I ask, as I try to work out where this conversation will end up, other than with the inevitable fact that I will say 'yes' to whatever is suggested.

'You know how our minister has been off sick for a while and the locum has left for the winter?'

'Yes.' Already I'm saying 'yes'!

'How would you feel about leading the services, you being educated and all that. You've been coming each Sunday anyway, haven't you?'

'Yes ... ' Again with the 'yes', why do I do that?

'Excellent, that's agreed then.'

'Ah! But I meant I was coming each Sunday, not that I ...'

'Nonsense, you'll be fine, we'll get things sorted,' she says with finality and then adds, 'Eileen of The Bu likes you fine and Willa agrees.'

'But I've hardly spoken to Eileen, or to Willa for that matter!'

'No, well, maybe not. But I was speaking to Eileen and Willa last week. They said Nessie and Ina were pleased with the way you looked after them,' she says. 'And Ann the Post says the boys are right polite when they come in for their comics from south.'

And so that's it, then. I've been selected, vetted, commissioned without me knowing anything about it. I had noticed that the men on the island were quiet; perhaps I understand a little about why now. From now on, I will be preaching each Sunday through the winter until the minister recovers or the locum returns in the summer. I think, perhaps, the travelling has not helped the minister's health. We don't have a minister on Eday but we share one with our neighbouring island. The service is at two o'clock, which allows the minister to take the service on Stronsay first at eleven o'clock then come over on a fishing boat to take our service. Some days that can be a thirty-minute sail and on others it may be as much as an hour or more. Over the years there have been many re-enactments of the scenes on the Sea of Galilee. The decision to sail or not is down to the skipper in charge of the boat and doesn't take account of the temerity or sea-worthiness of the minister. As a consequence, ministerial faith can be strengthened or broken by this sea crossing. There have been occasions where services on Eday were slightly delayed while the 'Restoration of the Reverend' took place at Tommy and Jenny's cottage prior to coming to the church. After really poor crossings the minister can take on a green tinge for the duration of the service and the prayers, heartfelt for salvation of body and soul, are intense but brief in the obviously swaying pulpit.

There's only one more question.

'When would you like me to start?'

'Well not straightaway, I'll have to speak again to the minister looking after us on the mainland. He says he'll send you his service for the week with his sermon. You must just read that to us since you're not trained – yet.'

Selected, vetted, commissioned and set up! And apparently waiting to be fully trained as well ...

'Let's say we get you started in a fortnight, would that suit you, Doctor? You'll not be going anywhere, will you,' she says, making more a statement than a question of it.

4

Hymns of the Heart

Two weeks later and I'm outside the church: a large stone-grey building that sits down tightly into the hillside, sheltering from the wind, like a solitary mountain hare. Once it would have welcomed hundreds of worshippers when, in times past, the island had over six hundred inhabitants. Push through the large blue-grey storm doors and you're into the small but immaculate vestibule. On each side are two golden-brown doors of combed lacquerwork, unchanged since they were hung years ago. Damp and greyness cling to the air, made worse by the tired winter light filtering in from somewhere high above. Continue left or right along the wood-panelled wall ahead, push open the felt padded swing doors and suddenly the whole place is bright with light streaming from the eight enormous plain glass windows that dominate the sanctuary. You've come under a choir gallery, and spread in front of you is row upon row of perfectly polished cedar pews, rich with history. There's easily seating for three hundred parishioners.

It's in this tidal flow of history that I must lead worship today and I'm very aware of this. What matters most is not the numbers of folk that come on each Sunday now but that we continue to spin the thread of island living, traced through time and woven into this special place. People will pass by on the road outside as we worship today and although they will only come in for funerals, they need to know this place still breathes. Three pins hold the island on the map and prevent the wind stripping it off into the North Sea. The church, the school and the surgery. Without these points firmly anchored, a vulnerability develops that nibbles at confidence, like a field mouse in winter on hot water pipe insulation. With that cooling effect, folks drift towards the warmth of security on the mainland.

After a brief word with Jenny and a quick check with Tommy, the organist, to make sure he has all the hymns sorted out, I walk slowly down the right-hand aisle and climb gingerly up to the pulpit. This is set at dizzying height and almost level with the choir gallery at the back of the building. I'm careful to close the little pulpit door to make sure I don't inadvertently plummet out, should I get overenthusiastic at any point. Nerves will prevent exuberance today.

Immediately below the pulpit I can see the top of Tommy's head as he sits at the old pedal harmonium. Shining red mahogany with five octaves of notes and two foot pedals to drive the bellows. The louder you play, the faster you must pump. Behind him are thirty rows of golden-yellow pews with the five people that make up the congregation sitting against the back wall. There are two reasons for folks sitting at the back. The first is a natural reticence to literally and metaphorically 'put themselves forward'. The second, more practical – it is warmer back there as the wooden panelling shields them from the draughts. There's no heating on in the church as it's not cold enough yet, being only November.

'Verily I say unto thee, inasmuch as ye did it not to one of the least of these, ye did it not to me ...'

Oh dear ...

'For where thou must aspire to dwell with the seraphim and cherubim ...'

I'm stuck with these words sent by post from the mainland minister, who, it appears, was born in 1853. Untrained in spiritual matters, the Church will not let me use my own words. This cautious approach to the use of words contrasts dramatically with the Health Board's approach to life, which was to appoint me to the 'island at the top of world' from an inner-city environment and let me get on with it. I don't understand the half of what this minister is trying to say so dear knows what the folks in the last pew will make of it. I must speak to Jenny and see what we can do about translating this archaic text into modern language. We may have to continue the thread of history but we could at least use new wool! Let's get on to a hymn quickly. I am allowed to choose these, so long as I stick to the hymnary and Tommy can play them.

Love divine, all loves excelling.
Joy of heaven to earth come down ...

Okay, that's a bit better but what is Tommy doing? There's a very small white sweet he seems to pop into his mouth before he starts each hymn and then lays carefully to the side of the keyboard once he's done. There's also a slight sheen coming from the top of his head towards the end of each hymn. There's no time to think about that just now. If I don't crack on and get through this stuff I won't be able to see to read it shortly.

One of the other reasons the service is at two o'clock in the afternoon and no later is the lack of winter light. There are magnificent gas lamps suspended from high in the ceiling, with two long chains hanging down from the gleaming white shades. Each chain has a little dog tag on them saying 'On' and 'Off' and these allow you to control the gas flow to the mantle. The lamps aren't used, though, because the gas is too expensive. This will be the last service in the church until spring now, si   we won't be able to see when the nights draw in further. Sunset will be just before three o'clock shortly. We'll transfer next week to the old manse, which unlike the church does have electricity, but I suspect will be no warmer as it sits in the damp hollow below the church. There's no point in using up good crofting land for something unproductive like a manse.

Final hymn now and Tommy is still swapping that sweet about while he coaxes the reluctant organ to give up its notes. I pronounce the benediction and carefully open the pulpit door while checking my parachute straps before descending to the ground. I'm sure the oxygen is thinner up there.

'Tommy! What is that sweet you keep sooking when you play the organ?'

'You gave it to me.'

'I did? When did I do that?'

'When you told me I had angina, you said I should sook the tablet before exercise. A field mouse has chewed a hole in the bellows of the old organ and even with me taping it up they still leak.'

'So you have to pedal harder to get it to play!'

'Yes, but if I keep sooking the tablet I get a headache, so I take it out at the end of each hymn. Besides, it's wasteful and if I'm careful I only need one tablet.'

'Tommy!'

'Yes, Doctor.'

'Come and see me at the surgery tomorrow and we'll see what we can do.'

The switch between roles catches me unawares. When I came into church to take the service it was clear the folks thought of me as 'minister' and yet immediately afterwards here I am as 'doctor' again. Come to think of it, I forgot I was 'doctor' when I was in the pulpit too. Otherwise, I would have realized sooner that Tommy's sweet was actually his GTN tablet for his angina.

Over the next few weeks I work with Tommy on his medication. I should really arrange an ECG and probably an exercise test on a treadmill to secure the diagnosis of angina. The first test would have to be done in Kirkwall and the second would need a trip to Aberdeen. Neither of these tests is really likely to change the way I manage Tommy's condition, so we invent a new test. The 'Pedal Organ Stress Test'. How many verses of a standard hymn can Tommy play before he begins to feel discomfort. At the end of our tests we're up to six full verses of 'Give Heed, My Heart' to the magnificent arrangement by J. S. Bach. It seemed appropriate for the test really.

5

The Sea Croft

Early December and it's completely dark in the morning now. At half past seven there isn't any glimmer of light through our bedroom window. Stretching out my hand to switch on the bedside light, there's time to lie back and breathe. Not a sound. No wind rustling the grasses, nothing disturbing the air to hint at coming gales. Nothing. Even the birds on the shore are silent. This is bliss. So different from the hectic pace of Glasgow, with the early commute to work and the endless queue of patients. Moving here seemed crazy a few months ago but now it's beginning to feel like one of the best decisions we've made.

Levering myself up to sit on the edge of the bed, the mattress edge sags, threatening to tip me off. I put my hand back on the pillow to steady myself. When I bring it back, black hairs tumble on to my legs and my palm is covered in thick strands that I just sit and stare at. Picking up the rootless hairs in my palm I play with them, bemused at where they've come from. Eventually, I look round at the pillow and see more hair lying in careless clumps where my head has been. My hand goes quickly to the back of my head, lifting off another handful of hair when I bring it forward again. There's no pain or tenderness or bleeding from my scalp, my hair is simply falling out. Running my hand over the back of my head there is the feeling of very fine stubble in some areas. Like velvet when you run your hand the wrong way on the pile. Shaking Maggie awake, I ask her to look at the back of my head.

'You have alopecia,' she says, yawning. 'You feeling okay otherwise?'

'I feel fine. Never felt better really ... was just thinking that when I woke up.'

'I'll have a proper look in the daylight. We'd better get the rascals up or we'll be late.'

I don't know if she deliberately doesn't give me any sympathy or realizes that it doesn't really help me, making me react angrily. I don't like it when my body doesn't work. It seems like an insult: a mechanic driving an old banger. I'm not bothered about my appearance, the hair should grow back with time. It's the fact that it should choose to fall out in the first place that bothers me. It feels like a weakness. The feeling driven by the knowledge that alopecia can appear after times of stress. I don't like to admit how difficult work was before we left Glasgow. I was on the edge of forgetting, letting the arguments with partners slip away as I settled into my own practice. The alopecia has brought those thoughts back to me. Into my escape to the island, the place I'm beginning to think of as home.

Down in the kitchen the room is warm with the heat from the Morsø stove. There's comfort in the red glow radiating through the thick glass of the doors. As a child I would sit for long periods looking into our brown glazed stove, opening the doors to watch the flames flickering in the fire-caves created as the coals burned away. The hottest flames deep in the caves, intensely blue and all-consuming. Purifying flames that I later learn sterilize and obliterate. Young as I was, I knew there were times when I needed to shut out the world. I would watch the flames, captured by the hypnotic boiling universes in the fire-caves that drew in my thoughts and cleared my mind. The memory of the childhood fires relaxes me again and I turn around to see how breakfast is progressing.

The boys are munching away at cornflakes. Martin and Matthew are tidily dressed but much to their delight not in school uniform; there's no point in a school of ten pupils. Murray is running around without a nappy in the vain hope that we might potty-train him soon.

'When are you going to finish that painting, Dad?' asks Matthew. 'That otter's tail isn't right.'

I've developed a fascination with otters, which I've been trying to find around the island. I can see their tracks and places where they lie up during the day, but I've never yet seen an otter. To compensate, the wall behind the fire has been coloured with pink heat-resistant paint (the only colour the shop had) and I've decorated it with two otters diving among seaweed, chasing each other around the black lacquered flue.

'I might get to it today. Do you think the tail should swing the other way?'

'I think so. It doesn't look like the ones I've seen in the books.'

Matthew is very keen on all kinds of animals and soaks up information on anything he sees. I agree to adjust the tail next time I work on the painting. At quarter to nine the Land Rover draws up and we send the boys off to school while I go through the dining room and open the surgery door. Outside it's barely light as I open the gate to the roadside and look up the hill. I'm not looking for patients now, I know they will come. I just like to remind myself where I am, feeling the air on my face and listening to the silence.

Morning surgery is a little different today as two mums have arrived for their antenatal checks. Both babies are due in the early spring and they will have to go into Kirkwall soon for a check-up by the consultant from Aberdeen. For the moment, though, I'll look after them. I quite like antenatal clinics, mostly because the patients are usually healthy and cheerful. Unlike the delivery of a baby, which is very surgical, antenatal care is quite medical and it suits me. There's a strange intimacy in the process of looking after someone's child while it remains hidden in the womb. Both of us, mother and doctor, are on the outside doing our best to make sure everything the baby needs is in place.

Mum feels the rumbles, the kicks, the little hiccups. Movements she's allowed herself to be wrapped round, while multiple tappings from inside tell her her baby is still there and growing.

I have to manage from the outside. Checking the baby's growth and the way it is lying needs a mixture of imagination and careful palpation of mum's abdomen. Discerning a head from a bottom sounds straightforward but bottoms can be particularly hard and cause confusion. During this process you make contact with a person inside a person, and I'm never quite sure what both parties make of being pushed around. Then there's a moment of closeness as I rest my ear on mum's tummy. The only way to hear the baby's heartbeat is to place the cone-shaped 'Pinard' directly on the mother's tummy and lay your ear against the flattened end of the cone. Somehow this feels intrusively close, different to when you look in a patient's ears and eyes with various scopes. There's a lingering amazement when I hear the minute bumps of the baby's heart too. A hundred and forty bumps a minute, fast and steady, heralding another life here on the island.

Both mums are well today, although I'm a little unsure about one baby, which seems small for the dates we have. It is lying high up in the womb, across the way instead of up and down. None of this is a definite sign of a problem but sometimes the placenta is low-lying and getting in the way of the baby, forcing it to lie sideways. She still has two months to go yet and so this fact is just worth noting for now and not something to worry us. I tell mum about what I find and mark '?Transverse?' on the maternity card, then we agree to wait and see what the consultant says next week when she's seen in Kirkwall.

I'm just about to call in the next patient when the phone rings. Reaching out, I indignantly brush more hairs from my sleeve before I pick up the receiver. Suddenly I'm aware that both mums would have seen the recent development of a bald patch on the back of my head. Perhaps I should have explained it but how do you explain latent stress?

'Malcolm, how are you settling in?' It's the Chief Medical Officer. 'You should be finding your feet now, I hope. I see you've only sent in one person to the clinic with back pain. Are you managing the rest of the patients yourself? Excellent. Listen, I wanted to make sure you were coming to the Area Medical Committee meeting next week – you know you're expected, don't you?' – and finally he pauses for breath.

'I read the letter, but I didn't think I could safely leave the island in case something happened.'

'Nonsense, we've made an agreement with the Health Board that all the doctors should attend the AMC. We fly you in and back the same day. If there is an emergency, then you'll go out with air ambulance and sort things out. Right then, see you next week.'

I'm both delighted and disconcerted at the end of this one-way conversation. Delighted because I've been trying to work out how to buy Christmas presents for the boys and a trip to Kirkwall will be just perfect for that. Disconcerted because I wasn't aware of being watched quite so closely. How did he know about the patient I had referred? Why would he care? It seems the small community effect isn't restricted to the island – it extends across the Health Board.

The next two patients come in together, as many of the husband and wife teams seem to do. Except Arthur and Lil aren't married, they are brother and sister. I haven't been able to get round everyone who is due a flu jab this year. Mostly because I forgot to order them in time, so the second batch has only just arrived. Arthur and Lil have come to make sure they have theirs before Christmas and visitors bring back infections from south. It wasn't something I'd considered but I suppose we are fairly protected from circulating viruses most of the year.

'The schoolchildren come back from the grammar school in Kirkwall for the holidays, Doctor, and there's always extra family visitors on the island too. We don't want to catch anything,' says Lil on behalf of them both.

'But the kids come back each Friday on the plane,' I say.

'Yes, but they stay on the farms mostly. Holidays, they're about the island more.'

I'm not sure about the logic but I'm interested in the concept.

'Are there other seasons when viruses are a problem?'

'Well, there's summer sickness. Usually about the end of May. They say there's something in the water. It happens most years, so we're used to it. It passes.'

Deciding to look into the water supply issue, I retrieve two flu vaccines from the fridge. It's quite difficult to get the vaccines out to the island while making sure they don't spoil. If the temperature rises too much during transport, then the vaccine efficacy falls dramatically. I had to make sure I picked them up straight away from the airstrip as soon as the plane landed, carefully taking the freezer bag they came in back to the surgery and putting the vaccines in the fridge again.

Just as they're leaving with two sore arms, Lil turns to say, 'Would you be good enough to visit Erland today, Doctor, please? He was going to come with us but isn't quite feeling up to it. We said we'd ask you to call. He's expecting you.'

Finishing the surgery, tidying away the antenatal cards and Pinard, I hesitate for a moment. Then picking up a fresh card, I take it through to the kitchen with me for coffee.

'What name do you want on your antenatal card, Maggie?' I ask as I walk into the kitchen.

'Do I need one yet? A card, not a name.'

'I think so, you'll have to go into Kirkwall for scans after Christmas. Do you want to be Mrs Alexander or Dr Simpson on the card?'

'I'll be Mrs Alexander, just like all the other times.'

'Okay. I'll get the card made out and we can do your booking bloods and such this week.'

Baby number five is on the way. There's nothing to worry about, as all the other pregnancies have gone pretty well. Maggie's asthma was difficult to manage in her first pregnancy, which made the birth complicated, but there weren't any obstetric issues. We very nearly didn't make it to hospital with our last baby, Little Murray, as we left things a bit too late. Several red lights were negotiated in the early hours of the morning.

After coffee I drive round to see Erland, popping a flu jab into my medical bag before I go. Finding his croft isn't as easy as I'd hoped, as there's no obvious road leading to the shore. By now, though, I know to look out for the telltale sign – closely cropped grass. An Orcadian signpost. I've recently bought a strimmer for the surgery to help me keep our roadside grass tidy too. At a break in the fence there's a long straight track leading to the sea with nothing else to indicate any habitation other than the carefully shorn grass. The grass is greener than the surrounding fields and has the appearance more of a lawn than the rough grazing in surrounding fields. I edge the car carefully down the track at first until I realize I needn't be so cautious. Just like visiting Ina, the surface is firm, solid with compacted stone that will never wash away or become muddy in the winter gales. Gradually driving westwards towards the sea, there's still no sight of a croft house, only the island of Faray in the distance.

Faray used to be inhabited and the croft houses can be seen still, scattered along the spine of the island. There was a reliance on sheep, which is where the name comes from – 'faer' meaning sheep and giving the island its correct pronunciation, 'Fayr-ay'. The road past our kitchen window is the Faray road and set still at the crossroads below the surgery is an old post box cut into a rickle of stones. This is the Faray post box – where, in days past, letters and packages for the island could be left. When weather and tide suited, the post would be taken from the shore just below Erland's by the postman in an open sailing boat across to the island.

After two hundred yards or more, the downward hill steepens slightly, then swings to the right, revealing a perfect croft sitting at the edge of a low cliff. The croft house itself is sheltered from the worst of the elements by outhouses and sheds corralling it protectively from the wind. The view is stunning across the water to Faray, with the low rolling hills of Rousay to the south-west. There's an openness to the view on this side of the island, an expanse of water and sky, with suggestions of the deeper ocean beyond. Westray Firth lies behind the sparseness of Faray and beyond it is the vast nothingness of the Atlantic. This shore is a place of the sea. Unlike other crofts, which are land-based, working the soils and peat bogs around them, this is a shore house. This is a sea croft, a place of creels and nets. Boat knousts – hollows to draw clinker-built wooden boats up safe from the tide – sit at the top of slipways cleared of stones. The smells are not the staleness of animals and fermenting grain but the freshness of salt and pungent seaweed. The air is not damp with straw and byres of urine, it is free of intrusive human or animal scent.

I knock on the door and let myself in. Erland is sitting in his sparse living room beside an unlit fire. Laying his *National Geographic* to one side, he motions me to the other seat, watching me quietly, sizing me up as he swings back and forth in his Orkney chair, always keeping the front legs slightly off the ground. The chair is a work of art in itself, crafted in pine, with the seat and high back made of oat straw ropework. The straw-work back wraps round him covering him to the shoulders, fitting perfectly, like the shell of a hermit crab, protecting him from the chill draughts that drive round the window frames.

As we talk about his difficulties with his Parkinson's disease, he lifts a bag of pandrops from the pocket of his knitted jacket, motioning me once again to take one. He is having more problems with the sudden freezing of his muscles that comes when the balance of medication isn't quite right. Conversation meanders from topic to topic – creel fishing, crofting, weather – until he appears to tire. Suddenly the Orkney chair is thrown backwards by what I think must be a muscle spasm, making me jump up to catch him. Until once again I see that recurrent Orcadian twinkle in his eye, as the top of the chair comes perfectly to rest against the bureau behind him. Balance perfectly restored. I have been caught, as so many others have, by his party piece.

After I've given him his flu jab, partly in retribution for him catching me out, he invites me to look round his sheds and outhouses. As much out of politeness as anything I agree, as I'm not sure what can be special about them. Entering the first shed, I expect the usual clutter of implements and boxes that are part of crofting. Instead, the shed is immaculate. Weak sunlight falls through the skylight high in the roof, picking out the browns and greys of the rafters worn with age but dry and sound. The roof space is free of cobwebs and dust. Beneath the rafters are two parallel stacks of peat, separated by a narrow passage the exact width of the wooden barrow by the doorway. The smell is indulgent, as the oils captured in each carefully placed peat are released to fill the shed. Erland flicks a switch by the door and the splendour of the whole enterprise is revealed. The floor, which is entirely dust-free, is accurately marked with a bright-white line delineating the limit of each stack. The line of each stack is exactly even, each peat in the stack jutting out at the same distance. Everything must be in its place. The dust and fragments of broken peat are gathered in a bucket near the door, ready to be dampened and packed into the fire in the evening before retiring to bed, keeping the fire smouldering through the night air.

As I drive reluctantly away from this sea haven, I'm left not knowing if I've been educated or warned. Was he showing me how things should be done in the neat precise manner of a seaman bachelor or was he showing me what I can never hope to achieve? I suspect it was a bit of both, the laying down of a challenge with an impossible mark to aim for. We'll see next year, when I cut the peats on our peat bank behind the house. He still never told me which of the three peat banks behind the house is mine.

6

Night Skies

London Airport. It always makes me smile that the folks here should have chosen that name for the airstrip. You wouldn't expect a group of red-painted wooden sheds to be called London Airport but here I am sitting outside them, waiting on my flight to Kirkwall and the Area Medical Committee meeting. There's the ever-present tension between tongue-in-cheek humour and cocking a snook at things regarded as flash from down south. The name is legitimate, though, as the airstrip lies on the narrow stretch of low-lying sandy soil between the Bay of London in the east and the Sands of Doomy in the west. I wouldn't put it past them to have called it Doomy Airport either.

There is just enough warmth in the low winter sun this morning to allow me to sit outside on the galvanized metal box in front of the main shed. Perhaps not the safest place to sit, as it contains the flares for marking out the runway for night flights. Beside me, the two mums I saw last week are chatting away about the antenatal clinic they have to attend, concerned in case the consultant decides they have to go to Aberdeen to have their babies. That may happen to one of them, I'm afraid. Maggie too will have to fly in shortly for her first scan, which I booked for her last week but that won't be done until after Christmas.

It's frowned on a little to look after your own family members, but the alternative is ludicrous, given the geography. Maggie would either have to sail to another island to see a GP or fly in to Kirkwall and back at considerable expense. So, we compromise. Last week I examined her thoroughly, took relevant booking bloods and urine samples, then completed all the forms. This took about half an hour instead of a whole day if she saw someone else, who would do exactly the same things. Maggie needs to trust me when I do this; even though we share the clinical decisions, she is still dependent on me actually carrying them out. I don't suppose everyone would be comfortable with this arrangement. We like the closeness it brings.

Once we're all strapped into the little ten-seater plane, it jolts us over the rough ground before we turn north into the wind and take off over Stennie Hill. Swinging west then south, I can just catch a glimpse of Mike and

Murray playing in the garden. I wave but neither of them looks up now they're used to the plane buzzing overhead.

Attending AMC meetings down south was mostly a necessary chore. A dreary drive accompanied by the usual parking hassle, only to end up in a nondescript city building of ancient corridors and tired meeting rooms. It was helpful to keep up with the local politics and to know about changes that may be happening but you could never call it inspiring. Here, it's entirely different. Where else are you allowed to fly to a meeting with a pilot who delights in making the plane skim low over the sea as you head for mainland? He takes us towards Egilsay, dipping the starboard wing down to let us see St Magnus's Church and then banks sharply over the waves, flying us south towards Shapinsay. Beneath us, huge Atlantic grey seals are hauled out on the grey-green seaweed-covered skerries and rocky outcrops. Frightened cormorants scatter from their rocky perches, necks outstretched as they fly fast and low over the wave tops, spooked by the sound of the twin propellers beating above them. I can't believe this excitement is part of my job as I watch the shadows shift and shape-change below me. Shadows that are long even towards midday, as the mid-winter sun barely prises itself over the southern hills before sinking again.

After we land, the three of us from Eday share the same taxi and chat on the way into town. I make sure to ask for pointers for shopping before we're dropped at the hospital. Following the two mums into the main entrance, I go over to the receptionists before going on my Christmas present hunt. Once they realize who I am, they wave me into their room. I want to say hello to the people who are my link to the outside world. I'm disappointed to find the thing I call 'Balfour Control' when I use the short-wave radio in the car is just a handset and a small grey box up on a shelf above the telephone exchange. I had hoped for something grander, more imposing, to give me confidence when I need to call for help. After a brief chat to the telephonist, I find the laboratory Portakabin behind the main hospital where I need to collect more blood sample bottles and bags for the surgery.

The lab is tiny, with silver-grey machines crammed on to the worktops. I don't know why I thought it would be bigger; it's not as if this is a big city hospital. I have a quick chat with Ian, who had told me all those months ago how to spin Ina's blood, then he shows me where to gather my supplies. Walking into town after my visit, I'm struck by how little equipment there is in the hospital. I thought it was just the island that was poorly resourced medically – with the exception of the centrifuge and that huge computer, everything else in the surgery is mine – but lots of the tests I thought would be carried out at the hospital have to be sent off to Aberdeen after the samples have been prepared.

The same cannot be said of Kirkwall which, in contrast to Eday and its single shop, seems like a metropolis crammed with an array of shops with all sorts of goods. Walking up Bridge Street from the harbour, I have to stop myself spending all my time in Scarth's hardware store, distracted like a child by all the tools, ironmongery, pots and pans. With only two weeks to go, my mission today is the boys' Christmas, not mine. The trick with Santa is to make the boys believe they are asking for the impossible when all the time that's exactly what he plans to bring. Not any different from other parents' difficulty, you might think. However, to heighten the excitement we don't write our letters to Santa until Christmas Eve, burning them in the fire and sending the messages in the smoke up the chimney to the North Pole. There have been nerve-racking moments in the past when at the last minute someone gets a new idea of what they want. That was hard enough when we had all the shops beside us. Now I have just one shot at getting it right. As I turn the corner into Albert Street, I see the place I was told about – Leonard's. A newsagent with the top floor given over entirely to toys, giving me plenty of choice.

After two hours of dashing about, I'm fully laden with packages and a large box carefully wrapped in thick brown paper to protect it from small prying eyes. Swapping the packages about from arm to arm as the muscles ache and complain alternately, I manage to make my way to the AMC meeting back at the Health Board. A meeting that turns out to be as mundane as those down south, and I leave with a clear impression that the main purpose was to make sure the island doctors hadn't completely lost touch with reality. A risk that seems entirely possible, given the various states of dress and manicure of my remote colleagues. I'm not sure catching up with everyone has helped either, as they all seem to be more confident about the job than I am. Some of them have to stay overnight in Kirkwall to wait on their flight home in the morning and this doesn't seem to worry them, apparently unconcerned that their island is without a doctor for all that time. When I ask them about this, they seem surprised I should give it a second thought. I'm not so comfortable and have been feeling all day that I'm in the wrong place. Like playing truant from school and spending the whole day concerned I would get caught. Despite being on the island for over three months now, being away doesn't feel like freedom. I'm only happy when once again the little plane takes off in the last of the afternoon light for the twenty-minute flight back home.

Before we came here I couldn't settle on islands. We used to stay for weekends on Maggie's home island of Bute in the Firth of Clyde and whenever the last ferry left for the night I was troubled by a sense of isolation. A feeling of entrapment that I wasn't able to shake off until morning and the boats started sailing again. I wonder if it's because I don't like being dictated to, forced into situations that I have no control over. It seems to me that islands dictate. There are limits to what they allow and one thing they don't allow readily is escape. The feelings are beginning to change a little now, though, and as the plane crops the heather hillside, grazing the West Side Road before landing, there's a settling of the concern I've felt all day. I'm back where I should be. Perhaps it's just the sense of responsibility that eases now I'm back, but it definitely feels better to be here.

When I get back to Heatherlea, I'm sent straight back out again to go and see Sue and Ken at 'Costa'. I had forgotten that we had agreed a few weeks ago to take half of a pig they were fattening for Christmas. The pig has now been dispatched and the clean half-carcass is waiting for us. As I let myself into their kitchen it is the smell that meets me first. The room is filled with the soapy taint of cold fat, which gets stronger as I cross to the table. I'm immediately reminded of university pathology classes, a thought I quickly put out of my mind as I remember we are supposed to eat this specimen. The half-animal is lying on its side, its skin scraped clean of the coarse hairs that cover it.

'How do you want it done, then?' asks Ken as he weighs up my demeanour at seeing the animal.

'Not sure. What do you usually do?'

'You want half the head as well?'

'I don't think Maggie would know what to do with it.' I'm sure he's testing me now.

'Right, I'll just do what we usually do. You get the bags and labels ready.'

I have to remember that although Ken knows how to do the butchering now, this wasn't anything he had done before they arrived here. Like everyone, he has had to learn through trial and error the best way to manage up here. As I watch him expertly dissect the pork, carefully taking as much meat as possible so there's no waste, I have a growing sense of appreciation of just how close to crofting we are. Even in the doctor's house we are dependent on the others around us. The interweaving of our lives is much more apparent. Basic things provided by people we know. After about an hour and a half I have a freezer-load of joints, chops and pork mince ready for the winter, and I return home triumphant that we have a good quantity of fresh meat.

'So, what do you expect me to do with all that?' says Maggie, deflating my triumph as I lay the many bags on the table.

'Honestly, I'm not sure. I hadn't realized just how big a pig was.'

'Get it in the freezer then, and we'll decide later on.'

Actually, it wasn't that difficult to use the store of pork. Maggie found a recipe for sausages without skins, grinding the bread and herbs together before shaping them into a respectable sausage shape. With those and a significant number of burgers, we were able to make the bacon cuts into very enjoyable child-friendly food. Christmas dinner was almost certainly going to be a joint of roast pork.

A few days later, around ten o'clock in the evening, the phone rings. This time my heart doesn't miss a beat, although it probably should have. Surprisingly, the voice on the line has a strong Northern Irish accent – not anyone local. In a slightly harsh Belfast accent he explains that he's sorry to bother me but he has just vomited blood and thought he may need a little help. I quickly agree and, discovering that he's staying in the caravan at the pier while some repairs are being done to the sea wall, I pick up my things from the surgery and drive down.

Outside, the night is one that would be quite impossible to see on the mainland, where the pollutant electric light obscures everything. Here, the black velvet sky is bright with stars that fall all the way to the horizon in every direction. Clouds floating low over the sea have their individuality illuminated from behind, making their edges phosphoresce in the deep blackness. Light captured from the just visible moon waiting behind the horizon, reflecting through the clouds. As I turn slowly down the hill at Backaland towards the pier, the cream moon eases behind the holms in the east, picking out the single remaining house in the moonlight and suspending it briefly on the sea surface before allowing it to sink again into the darkness.

Once I find Mick – he really is called that – lying on the couch at the front of the caravan, he manages a half-smile and then curls up again, clearly in a lot of pain. Careful examination shows he almost certainly has an ulcer which has bled. The cause of this is visible in the remains of the liquid refreshment scattered around the caravan. Normal practice is to admit patients like Mick to hospital under the care of the surgeons, who can intervene if things get worse. At present, apart from his pain, which is obviously severe, he is in remarkably good shape, which presents me with a dilemma.

Imagine what it would be like to fly through a night like this over a sea sparkling in the moonlight. Looking down, watching the lights of crofts and farms twinkle below as you fly in at two hundred feet around each island. A honeytrap, waiting for the romanticism of the remote life of a country doctor to cloud your judgement. Making you forget to balance all the risks while you're distracted by the scenery. Night flying has always been more difficult than in daylight. Of course, there are instruments on the little planes to fly by, but much of the skill in landing on a remote airstrip is visual. The grassy strips are nuanced, shaded differently by the light of the moon or invisible in moonless blackness when they are picked out solely by the light of a few flares roughly marking the limits of the grass. The hidden rising and falling of the ground unexpectedly affects the response from the plane. Only pilots experienced in each individual strip are allowed to land on them at night.

The other side of my dilemma is diagnostic. What exactly am I dealing with? Probably an ulcer but there are other conditions, too, that mimic the symptoms and others that may occur in parallel. Some of these I would test for if we were in hospital but to do any of these things now I need to arrange a night air ambulance flight. My final decision is made by the weather, always the weather. Stable conditions tonight mean I can fly my patient at any point if I need to so I can take a little time and try a newer treatment. Medication is used to treat ulcers routinely now but hasn't been used to treat potentially bleeding ulcers outside hospital as far as I know. I'll have to trust myself and see how things go.

Explaining to Mick what I'm going to try, he's happy not to be admitted to hospital. Loading him with my chosen treatment, using more than usual doses, I leave him with strict instructions to call me if things change and drive back to the house. Even in the short time I've been with Mick in the caravan the night has changed. The magic has drained from the sky as the moon rises and washes the black sky in pale light. It's still beautiful, still peaceful, but without the intensity of earlier. A tawny owl floats briefly across the windscreen as the car climbs the hill from the airstrip I hope not to use tonight, if my judgement is correct.

Back at the house, I chat briefly to Maggie before she goes up to bed and I settle by the little stove in the kitchen again to read for a while. I'll go back down to the pier at one o'clock in the morning to see my patient again, just to be sure. I won't sleep anyway until I know my treatment has a chance of working. A little more coal goes on the fire – peat burns too quickly to keep the stove in overnight – as I open my next book on whales but I'm not ready to read just yet. What did Dr MacKenzie do when he was waiting through the night? He always seemed so confident when he visited us. Was he? His hospitals were twenty miles away by road and sometimes in the winter we were cut off for days by snowfall. Here, I can call a military helicopter if I get approval or I can ask the lifeboat to come out. Dr MacKenzie must have had times where he had nothing to do but wait. I wonder if he prayed? I don't remember seeing him in church when I went as a child. Is confidence an illusion we create as doctors, necessary but unreal, lacking in foundation? How do we know when a doctor is not waving but drowning? It's not something we ever speak about when we're together as a group. The others at the AMC meeting seemed confident, almost blasé, when they spoke about their islands. I don't feel that way. Life here feels like taking a continual risk.

In the morning I'm much less uncertain. Mick was already feeling better when I saw him again through the night and had no further bleeding. I went to see him before breakfast and took some bloods, so I can get results today if I need to change anything in his treatment. I particularly want to know if he has an inflamed pancreas as well as his ulcer, as that will need a different approach.

I'm on my way back down to the pier now as it's Wednesday again, an event which seems to come around quite quickly now. I spotted the MV *Islander* from the schoolroom window coming down Eday Sound on its way to us from Westray. This week's school lesson was cut short to let me get to the pier on time. When I started taking the services in the church the school teacher, who wasn't religious, obviously took note and tackled me in the shop one day. Could I teach the class Religious Education on a weekly basis? It would have to cover other religions as well as Christianity. Would I be able to do that?

Well, that seemed like a challenge, so today we finished a lesson on the Far Eastern religion of Shinto. Probably more properly called the practice of Shinto, as it is as much a tradition as a religion. At the time when the Vikings were beginning to come to Orkney, the practice of Shinto worship was being described in Japan. I was perhaps a little ambitious today when we tried to make *haraegushi* out of paper and then wave them about to purify ourselves. Once we'd completed these paper sticks, with streamers flowing from them, the class deteriorated into something that looked more like a Viking raid rather than a religious ceremony. Fortunately, I spotted the boat coming and hurriedly left the battlefield before things got worse.

The usual organized chaos reigns when I get to the pier. There is a pallet piled with Christmas trees just swinging off the boat, Stan's old Bedford is being loaded with animal feed by the forklift truck, people are waiting about for their boxes and crates to arrive. I've a few more small presents coming out from Kirkwall I want to hide before the boys come home from school and the weekly pharmacy supplies to pick up. The boat times will be different over Christmas and New Year, so I've tried to overstock a bit to see me through to January. The scene is quite different from the beauty and peace of last night, as a fog fills the sound between the islands. I hadn't thought about fog last night when I decided not to fly my patient out. Nothing is predictable here. I was going to pop in on Mick again, but I see he's working down at the sea wall. I'm not sure he should be doing that just yet, so I'll go and waste my breath and tell him.

7

Windstorm

Saturday morning and, with just over a week until Christmas, one of the fishermen calls from the pier telephone box to say they have a dog with a fish hook stuck in its nose. Can I do anything? I have no idea. When they arrive at the surgery I'm even less sure. The large black Labrador comes in through the gate happily wagging her tail and sporting a less than fetching piercing.

'What happened?'

'Ah, she was messing about in the fish boxes, Doc, and got hooked on the line that was lying among them.'

'I'm not really supposed to treat animals.'

'Aye, I know, but we'd have to take a day to go into Kirkwall with the boat to get her to a vet. Take a look anyway, will you?'

The hook is a large steel one used for line-caught cod and pollock. The point and most of its curved end is firmly embedded in the shiny blackness of the dog's nose. She's a patient animal, who lets me look carefully at the hook, moving it about a little to see what pain, if any, it causes her. She's not happy. To take the hook out I'm going to have to push it through the cartilage and then cut off the point and barb. Exactly the same way I would deal with a deeply embedded hook in a fisherman. With a fisherman I can do a nerve block and freeze the affected area; all I know about dogs is there are a lot of nerves in their nose. Deciding discretion is the better part of valour, I phone the vet in Kirkwall. I need to speak to him anyway about our geese, one of which is losing weight dramatically. After a ten-minute chat we decide I can try to anaesthetize the cartilage of the dog's nose with some local anaesthetic and see if the hook will shift.

Looking at the peaceful Labrador's nose was fairly straightforward, sticking a needle into it isn't something she was prepared to allow readily. Holding her as firmly as we can without hurting her, I make my first and only attempt. The needle on my syringe won't even go into the cartilage, there's no way I can push the plunger and inject the local anaesthetic. I had no idea that dogs' noses were so tough. No wonder they poke them into places with impunity. Before we distress the dog any more, I admit defeat.

'Sorry boys, you'll have to take her into Kirkwall, I'm afraid. She'll need to be knocked out to get that shifted.'

'Okay, Doc, thanks for trying.'

'Can you bring me back medicine for the geese while you're in? The vet said he'd leave some out for me.'

With that, the relieved dog leaps into the back of the pickup truck and they drive off. It hadn't occurred to me that I would be asked to look at animals too. I suppose I'm the nearest thing to a vet out here. The problem is that although vets are allowed to treat humans in an emergency, doctors aren't allowed to treat animals. Which is probably just as well, really, given that many of the medicines we use are not suitable for animals. If penicillin was tested today for human use it would never pass the safety checks. Even small doses are lethal for rats, one of the animals used to mimic human metabolism during the testing phase. I only found this out when a hamster we had needed antibiotic and the vet gave it oxytetracycline instead of penicillin. Deciding to stick to the animal I know for as long as I can, I gather the Christmas tree from beside the garage where Stan left it and take it into the house.

'Are we putting it up now, Dad?'

'Yep, shift the telly across a bit and we'll put it in that corner. Martin, go and get a bucket from the shed and fill it with coal.'

'I'sh know what I want for Chr'shmas,' says Little Murray with his distinctive lisp. 'I'sh want a cowboy suit and guns.'

This is definitely not the time to panic. There are five shopping days left and none of the parcels I brought back from Kirkwall has anything remotely like a cowboy suit.

'Oh really. That would be pretty good, wouldn't it? Do you think Santa will have one?'

'He has everything.'

He may be supposed to have everything but I'm not sure they make cowboy suits for the under twos. They do make red and cream sit-on wheelie horses, which was one of the parcels making my arms ache last week. Time to start the campaign.

'I bet he even has a horse you could sit on and charge at people.'

'I'sh want a cowboy suit and guns.'

Round one goes to Murray as we continue to decorate the tree and hang streamers and paper chains around the house and surgery. With Christmas coming, there's a steady stream of parcels arriving each morning with the post. The postman always hesitates at the garden gate, waiting for one of us to come out before he hands the parcels over, keeping prying eyes away from them as they're put into the garage instead of the house. The boys' comics arrive from Aunty Betty, posted faithfully each week, making sure she keeps in touch with them. The *Beano* this week has the twelve days of Christmas as demonstrated by Dennis the Menace and Gnasher. I'm never sure if it's me or the boys that enjoy the comics the most.

There are regular phone calls too, from friends and family, all of whom are becoming concerned about the weather. Are we surviving okay? The wind has been terrible down south. Are we sure we're okay? Actually, the weather is fine and still fairly warm, given it's December. We need coats and hats, but we've been out playing in the garden a fair bit. The medicine arrived from the vet today after the fishermen went into Kirkwall with the decorated dog. I've to give each goose 5ml of the worming liquid today and tomorrow. Deciding the only way this was going to happen was by soaking bread with the solution, I set off with my medication. Accurately measuring the dose on to the bread was straightforward; getting each goose to take only its measured dose wasn't. Albert, the dominant grey goose, has clearly had a little more than his fair share but hey, what's the worst that can happen?

Looking out the window the next day, Amelia, the snow-white goose, and Humphrey, the cross-eyed China goose, are grazing steadily on the grass. Albert isn't. Albert isn't doing much really, other than trying to stand. I watch him for the next ten minutes while I sip my coffee; he gives a great impression of a drunken sailor trying to cross a motorway. The comic effect is enhanced by him failing to control not only his legs but also his long neck, which is spiralling round as he staggers across the garden. There's nothing I can do for him as, unfortunately, in his greed he has overdosed himself with the medication. He'll just have to wait for the effects to wear off. It is a reminder to stick at what I know best, though. There is also the possibility he will appear in a future sermon once I get a freer hand with the content.

Finally, after a long week of waiting, Christmas Eve night is here and four small boys are busy constructing their letters to Santa. I've managed to manoeuvre the three older boys into asking for a Scalextric set. Something that is clearly impossible to get out here especially as 'we've' only just decided that's what 'they' want. We've even made it more impossible by deciding on the colour of the cars they will get.

'Right then, young Murray, let's help you with your letter. What have you written there?' I ask, looking at the series of squiggles that are his letter.

'I'sh want a cowboy set and guns!'

'Oh really, what about the horse you said you wanted last night?'

'Oh, I'sh still want that ... but I'sh need guns too.'

'Ah, right then ... Okay, let's put all that down but I'm not sure Santa will have room for it all on his sledge.'

The letters are duly completed and all four are placed one at a time into the Morsø stove and allowed to burn away, sending the smoke spiralling north to the Pole. Carrots, mince pies and milk are carefully placed on the hearth behind the fireguard, so the dog doesn't eat them prematurely, and four boys are tucked up in bed once more to wait like every other child for Christmas morning.

Fortunately, none of our boys are early risers so there's just a hint of daylight when ...

'Hands up, Dad, or I'sh will fire,' as Murray pokes a six-shooter up my left nostril, ready to pull the trigger. 'I'sh told you they would come.'

It is just as well the local shop has a Christmas gift room set up in the three weeks before the event. I spotted the set of guns and a cowboy hat when I was in for our bread supplies this week. The Santa magic survives another year.

'Dad, one of Santa's reindeer has broken the decorations with its antler.'

'And there's a sooty footprint in the hearth.'

'There'sh straw everywhere too, Dad. Bang. Bang, Bang.'

Maggie turns over in bed and smiles at me.

After the mayhem of Christmas morning has passed, Maggie sends the boys outside to play – me included – so she can begin to get the Christmas dinner of roast pork organized. As well as the Scalextric set there's a new red Frisbee to play with in the paddock where we think we might keep goats in the spring. Needing only jumpers to keep us warm, all five boys range over the paddock, chasing the recalcitrant Frisbee. Little

Murray is as good as the rest of us, managing to keep the disc flat as it flies through the air. Suddenly, an unexpected gust of wind lifts it high, taking the Frisbee soaring over the wall across the road into Millbounds' field. Scrambling over the drystane dyke, searching around the old cottage that stands ruined across from Heatherlea, I'm reminded of a shepherdess called Jenny Armstrong, who lived at the bottom of the narrow road opposite my childhood home. On one of the few times she left her native Carlops, a much younger Jenny had lived in the now ruined house opposite us, spending the summer tending sheep.

Latterly, sadly, she was confined to a wheelchair in the cottage she had lived in nearly all her life, a hardening of the arteries meaning both of her legs had to be amputated. She was in the Royal Infirmary in Edinburgh for the operations when I was a final year student and she was beginning to lose heart. After several months of hospitalization, she sorely missed her faithful sheepdog, Laddie. Laddie and Jenny needed no words to understand each other, they simply knew. Knew when it was time to feed the sheep, time to round up the faraway hens, time to gather the 'in-byre' flock of chickens. Knew when to stand still at a gate until the sheep had moved by, knew when to move slightly to keep a wanderer in line. Both watching each other all the time. I remember when, with only a single word, Jenny would send Laddie to gather in sticks for the Rayburn, returning to place them carefully in the hearth.

I popped in to see her one day, lying in her convalescence in the old-fashioned Nightingale ward on the first floor of the Infirmary building. The full splendour of the Victorian surroundings dwarfed Jenny as she lay curled up in the starched whiteness of her hospital bed. She was pleasant as ever but even quieter than usual, feeling that maybe she shouldn't go on. Each day she seemed to vacillate between determination to get home and despair at losing her mobility, her independence. None of the doctors looking after her thought she should even try to go home. I spoke to Sister on the way out of the ward and we agreed on a plan.

Two evenings later, after visiting hours and any danger of consultant appearances were passed, two human figures climbed the steps outside the Infirmary. Swinging open the doors under the carved entrance signs which said, 'I was sick and ye visited me' and 'I was a stranger and ye took me in', eight feet made their way quickly along the corridors and up the stairs to the ward. A very strange but well-behaved visitor slipped past Sister's door with nothing more than a quiet nod and smile from me. Jenny's face when she saw Laddie was worth all the subterfuge in getting her sheepdog into this animal-free environment. Whether it was the visit from Laddie or simply that Jenny decided enough was enough, from then on she was even more determined to get home on her own, refusing any thoughts of going into care. I visited her once or twice on the few days I was home after starting my junior hospital jobs and found her spinning her wheelchair about in the tiny cottage. Laddie stayed with friends now, though, and the faraway hens had been let go.

After an hour of playing outside and another good while setting up the Scalextric track, we sit down to a Christmas dinner that is one of the tastiest I have had in a long time. I suppose I've never really had farm-reared pork this fresh before. Having eaten more crispy crackling than I thought was possible, I settle by the peat fire in the living room to let the rest of the day slip away. Maggie is on the phone to her mum and the boys have finally given in and gone to bed. I may need to keep an eye on the fire though, as my pyromaniac tendencies seem to be to the fore again. Peat, good black peat, can burn really fiercely in a good fire. It can also burn quite fiercely in the chimney, as the oils coat the flue, creating sticky crusts that light in the updraught. No matter, I'll pour myself another whisky just to make sure the fire is well and truly under control before I go to bed. Most of the locals think I'm teetotal since they've never seen me in the pub or having a drink at a dance. It's probably as well to keep them thinking that way too.

Before Christmas I had a spell of calls through the late evenings to go and assist some drivers who had

had accidents in their cars on the way home, their cars slipping gently from the roads into the peaty ditches. No one was ever hurt but it was a good way of getting a lift home from the doctor. Eventually, I got fed up of this and it finally occurred to me what to do. As the first medical practitioner at the scene of a road traffic accident I have two things I can do after assisting any casualties. Firstly, I can bill the driver's insurance company for an emergency care fee and, secondly, I'm duty-bound to let the local police know that there has been an accident. Once I made these facts known to the next caller who requested my assistance, there didn't seem to be any more phone calls.

Two weeks into the new year and finally morning surgeries are not accompanied by the thud of Scalextric cars on the dining-room door. We've set the track up on the dining table, but the cars flying round the curves often completely fail to take the bends and wipe themselves out on the dining-room door. School has started again, and the normal weekly rhythm is established. Or at least it should be but today there doesn't seem to be anyone coming to the surgery. Wednesday morning is usually quite busy as folks drop in before the boat arrives and the shop goes full swing. Today there's no one. I wasn't bothered until sitting at my desk I realized there was no traffic on the road either. Nothing was moving. Giving up on surgery at ten o'clock, I set out on my rounds, pushing any further thoughts of absent cars away until I pass the shop. There are no cars at the shop either. I need fuel anyway so pull in at the pumps and start to fill up. Then I see two men in dark clothing standing slightly out of view around the corner of the shop. Their black and white chequered police hats are just visible.

'When did they arrive?' I ask when I go in to pay for the petrol.

'Came out this morning on the plane. Had to be today, there's a gale of wind due tomorrow.'

'I know Steven said it might be breezy. So, it's the police that have cleared the road?'

'Aye, it's not long before word gets around that they're here to check the road tax and insurance. We didn't tell you, though, you being official and all. We knew your car would be fine, Doc!' It's a statement that seems like a double-edged sword. 'One of us' but not.

Driving off up the road after a brief chat with the policemen, who again already knew who I was, it strikes me that my duty to inform insurers and the police after an accident must have brought consternation to quite a few folks on the island. The roads remain wonderfully quiet all day until the afternoon plane leaves. There is more traffic on the road throughout the evening than there has been all day. The movement only settles when we go to bed, as the sound of the rising wind murmurs in the chimneys.

Slowly the sound breaks into my sleep. A growl now, reverberating through the bedroom, coming up through the floor and causing the bed to vibrate, as if someone has clamped a giant engine to the side of the surgery beneath us that is making the whole house shudder. Looking up at the flat roof above our bed, it appears to be rising and falling.

'Are you awake, Maggie?

'Been awake for an hour, I was just letting you sleep.'

'Is the ceiling moving?'

'I think so. There's water pouring down the wall over there.'

Standing at the bottom of the bed I can just reach the low ceiling if I stretch. When I put my hand up, the ceiling moves up and down, away from my fingertips, rising by four or five inches each time. Each solid thump of the wind against the building sucks the roof up before releasing it again. The wind isn't blowing; there's nothing gentle about this wind. It is physical, alive and beast-like, pushing everything before it. It doesn't gust, it drives into, over, through the centre of you. At the moment it's trying to drive into and through our house. Water continues to run down the inside of our bedroom wall while the wind tries to prise the roof off and get in.

'Should we move?'

'I think so. We'll go through to the spare bedroom and shut this door just in case.'

Before leaving the bedroom, I can't resist looking out the window into the night. There is nothing to see but blackness and salt spray on the glass. The panes themselves are moving, flexing with the pressure of the wind, making the reflection of the room shrink and expand like those crazy mirrors at old-fashioned funfairs. Grabbing the bedding, we move through to the other side of the house, checking on the boys as we go. Even with all the noise around them, they're tucked up and sound asleep.

We both lie wide awake for a long time, listening to the wind as it attempts to rip the slates from the pitched roof above us. The slates clatter and argue with the wind as they cling to the sarking, waves of sound crossing the roof from end to end like spoons on a washboard or a manic football rattle. Even in this more solid part of the house, there's a shudder through the bed still as each lump of wind crashes against the building.

By six o'clock in the morning there's no point in trying to sleep and I get up to go down to the kitchen. The little stove is nearly out, the wind drawing the air through the spinners even though they are closed, the night's coal burned away. Riddling out the ash, I can hear the wind thirty feet above us, sucking across the top of the chimney. Rescuing the remaining embers, I re-stoke the fire, closing the door firmly. I open the spinners just a fraction to allow a little air to draw the flames and then go upstairs to the bathroom.

I hadn't realized that black lacquered flue pipe could become near see-through but that is what has happened in the five minutes I've been upstairs. The normally shiny black stove pipe is fiery red when I come back down, as the wind sucks fire up the chimney, pulling and gasping the air through the tiny opening in the spinners. Grabbing the oven gloves from the cooker, I screw the spinners tightly shut and force the handle of the door down as firmly as I can. Then I cross my fingers and hope that's enough.

Over the next twenty minutes the redness slowly subsides, leaving a lingering smell of hot metal in the room, the sooty glass on the doors burned clean in the updraught. Listening to the wind outside, there's no sign of any let up. I need to go outside for coal and to check the sheds now, before the day starts properly. I put my hand on the new door handle Steven had fitted and try to pull the door towards me. It doesn't come, stubbornly refusing to move. It should move, it's a new door after the old blue one, porous and peeling, finally disintegrated in November and was replaced. Putting all my strength into hauling on the handle, I manage to ease the door open a fraction before the wind thumps into the house again, sucking the whole thing out of my hands and slamming it shut. After several attempts I give up and go around to the surgery door, which fortunately opens more readily, sheltered as it is by the yard wall.

I've never experienced wind like this. A ferocious

anger driving solid punches of air into me from all sides. You can't lean into this fury, as it wrestles with you, thumping you from side to side. Unless I stay tight to the wall, the assault will succeed and knock me to the ground. Finally, I manage to get into the garage through the side door. Inside, the unconcerned rabbit is snug in its hutch, munching away on an old carrot while the gale rages around it. The wind sounds different in here, hissing through all the cracks and gaps in the planking, shaking the front doors and clattering the bolts, even with the car parked hard against them. There's no way to open them now without losing the roof. Steven warned me yesterday that there was a 'bit of a breeze' coming and that I should back the car against the outside of the garage doors. That way, I could get into the car if I needed to go out. Dust is swirling around in little tornadoes, spinning across the floor before collapsing on to it, only to be picked up and danced round again. Filling the bucket with coal, I beat a careful retreat into the house.

The boys are hopeful that school will be closed today and are reluctant to get ready, dragging out breakfast for as long as possible. They're out of luck when, as I suspected, the Land Rover draws up punctually at a quarter to nine. Holding them under the arms, we go one at a time from the surgery door to the back of the Land Rover and pile them in. Their neatly brushed hair and carefully adjusted hoods are blown to bits long before we get there. Retreating to the kitchen once they're gone, I look out the window towards the peat hill before going through to start surgery. When we arrived, I built a very heavy duck shelter out of three sheets of corrugated iron and a solid wooden frame. No more than two feet high, I expected this ground-hugging model to be immune to the wind. I was wrong, as I'm just in time to see this rise from behind the drystane dyke like the Tardis from *Doctor Who*. Rotating slowly in the air, it gyrates past the window, rising all the time, and disappears over the garage. Sprinting to the other window, I watch it clear the garage and thankfully the car, as it ends its journey over the wall in the field beyond the road. Another sprint through to the living room to see if I can see the ducks – who, it turns out, are happily puddling about beneath the bushes, having abandoned their shelter at dawn. The geese are tucked in behind the wall asleep, heads curled up under their wings. I seem to be the only one perturbed by the weather.

To try to improve confidentiality in the waiting room we've put a little transistor radio on the window ledge. Turning it on at nine o'clock, Radio Orkney's news and weather summary is just finishing with the comment that wind speeds on Fair Isle (forty miles to the north of us) hit a record 125 mph in the early hours of the morning. I don't feel quite so bad about my concern now.

Morning surgery is delayed by the quantity of water I

find in the consulting room, which has streamed down the wall during the night. The wind has been unsuccessful, so far, at peeling off the roof, although it's still having a good try. Ten past nine and, with wind speeds probably still around 80 mph, Jenny comes into the surgery for her monthly check-up. Her wig is held firmly in place by a scarf tied tightly under her chin.

'That was a black grass blow last night, Doctor. How did you get along?'

'Apart from the roof trying to leave, that duck shed actually leaving and water pouring down the wall, we're fine, Jenny. What's a grass blackener?'

'Well, it's only a proper gale when the grass goes black,' she says. 'Look out at the fields and you'll see what I mean. Will your wife be at the Guild this afternoon? We'll be on at two o'clock as usual.'

'I'll let her know.'

I had no idea what she meant about the grass until after the surgery. Crossing the road to see where the duck shed had landed, I manage to poke my head above the wall. In front of me the normally green and brown hillside is nearly black with battered and bruised grasses. The wind has whipped and flattened them so much the field is a dark green, dark enough to be taken as black. The rage of the storm is vicious, railing at everything in its path. Turning back to the surgery, I see the outside of the house for the first time, spattered with grasses and seaweed from the assault, even though we are half a mile inland.

The wind continues to blow for two more days, rarely easing or changing direction. They say it's only a south-easterly that digs in like that, venting its fury unremittingly, scarifying the island and pounding the beaches, ripping and tearing at the seabed as well. Huge piles of tangles are driven up on Warness Beach, the thick roots of kelp dragged from the sea bottom and thrown on to the sand.

After three days of unrelenting wind, great steam trains of air that roll through the island, quite suddenly there's silence.

Nothing.

A soundless cocoon settles round Eday, wrapping it up, soothing it after the brutality of the wind. Opening the yard gate before surgery as usual, I walk a little way down the road to the Faray post box and stand looking. A thin, dishevelled light seeps into the sky, giving the clouds and the battered hillsides a ghostly look in the aftermath of the storm. Yellow, like a bruise coming to the surface as the injured blackness gradually subsides.

Still there is silence. Turning slowly to try to pick up some scrap of sound, listening for a crack in the shell of the cocoon, the merest whisper, there is nothing. The island is stunned.

There's no sadness in this silence, just a sense of waiting, almost a dignity in the unmoving countryside refusing to be rushed into spurious activity. The storm is a fact, something inevitable, compulsory to life up here. Not to be fought against but endured, then put aside. Recovery isn't necessary as, apart from the cosmetic effects, there is no real damage anywhere. Sheds, byres, houses are all intact, the people used to living with the inevitable, planning for it each year. As I watch the landscape rest in the exhausted morning light, there's a feeling of being part of the island now. Having endured our first storm, a sense of acceptance develops between us, me and the island. I'm not trapped now, as I don't want to be anywhere else.

Then, imperceptibly at first, from the far end of the Faray Road the sound of a tractor chops through the silence, breaking into the quietness and prising open the cocoon. The chugging of the old engine as it coughs its way up the hill from Cusebay restarts the soundscape as today's work begins again on the island.

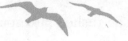

8

A Seal's Fate

Now the island is quiet again, the sound of the seashore, the piping of oystercatchers, the liquid call of the curlew, the hiss of the waves on the sand, all flow in through the bedroom window. The sound has become reassuring, a nightwatchman's call that all is well. During the day, I like to wander down to the shore to see for myself the setting for the nightwatchman sounds. Being on my own, standing at the edge of the island, where the land finishes and the rest of the world begins, has become a gathering place for me. A place where I can rest and collect my thoughts, a place to let my anxiety drift into the wilderness of the sea. Listening to the rhythm of the waves on the sand soothes me, sea breezes on my face refresh me.

Resting at the edge of the sea, watching it tug restlessly at the island shore, I can imagine all the life beneath the ripples and splashes of the lapping waves. Beneath those risings and fallings lie millions of creatures which easily move about the ocean. Am I envious of them? Envious of their ability to live and move freely in the depths of the sea? No, my envy is reserved for the bird I've come to see: its languid, lazy flight contrasting with sudden halts, hovering over the waves then plunging, diving down into the sea. My bird. Apparently relaxed and easy-going at one moment then immediately alert, focussed, considering before acting decisively. A change of mood only possible due to the spring of anxiety coiled constantly beneath the surface. An ice-white sea swallow, with sharp, blood-red beak and black 'judge's sentence cap' on its head. The name suggests freedom and exotic places. Arctic terns, with their delicate swallow tails and graceful undulating flight, have the ability to travel huge distances over land and sea. Imagine being able to connect Mill Bay, lying just below Heatherlea, with Matthews Island in South Orkney Islands. To fly from 59 degrees north to 60 degrees south then come back again. This sea swallow dipping into the waves in front of me will fish in the Weddell Sea in Antarctica this winter, a round trip of 45,000 miles. I envy its freedom.

Walking across the bay at low tide, I must be careful not to stand on the fishing line Willick has stretched through the sand. Thin, almost invisible, nylon buried beneath the sand, a large stone weighting down one end while the other is anchored to the shore just above the tideline. Every two yards or so, tiny baited hooks lie on the surface, waiting for their catch. As the tide creeps in across the sandy shingle, flounders move from the deeper water into the fertile bay, hoovering up tiny crustaceans and worms disturbed by the waves. Some of them will never return, held by the tiny hooks in the sand, anchored to the island. Getting close to the island can be rewarding and dangerous simultaneously.

The beat of the waves, the changing light, the wind singing through grasses, whistling over an iron gate, is beginning to absorb me, to pull against my restlessness and my need to control events. My need to make everything as good as it can be for those around me, family and patients. The dangers too are falling into perspective, the effect of isolation proving no different here than it was in the middle of the city. Sudden illness can strike at any moment. Here, I've transferred a heart-attack patient into the Coronary Care Unit faster than I managed in inner-city Glasgow.

I was savouring an afternoon coffee with Maggie, chatting about the ease with which I can transport patients from the island, weather permitting of course, when the phone rang. It was David, the assistant harbour master.

'Hi, Doc, we've a small problem we hope you can help with.'

'I'll do what I can.' Often non-medical problems are

set up this way; we've looked after a number of animals already and I'm wary of what's coming.

'There's a seal stuck in the inner harbour, the Simpson boys spotted it hauled out on the little beach. They think it's sick.'

'Isn't there a seal rescue centre on the mainland, David? What did they say? Have you called?'

'Yep, we called them and they're happy to come and get it ...'

'Well, that's perfect!' I cut in quickly, hoping to avoid an encounter with seal teeth, which I know all about from injuries to fishermen's hands.

'They're happy to come tomorrow and get it,' he goes on, ignoring me. 'There's a storm coming in fast this afternoon and they can't get out and back to mainland in time.'

Although I pretend otherwise, these non-human episodes are quite enjoyable really. Perhaps there's a little less stress in looking after an animal with no human companion. Anyway, a new puzzle to solve is always good and I try to think through what we'll need as we prepare a straw bed in the little shed between the house and the garage. This is rapidly becoming a hospital shed for sick animals.

When I get to the pier, word of mouth has ensured a small crowd has gathered to see what the doctor is going to do with this problem. And to give advice:

'Aye, Doc, you've a slippery problem there!'

'Do we need the police too? There's something fishy about this!'

'Are you going to "seal" its fate, Doc?'

'Always approach the blunt end first, Doc!'

Thanks, team! Sometimes it feels as though I'm the only entertainment on this island. Before diving in to see the potential patient, I hover on the harbour wall, scanning the sea for signs of other seals but this one seems to be completely alone. Separated from all its family members, it's found sanctuary on the little beach in the inner harbour for now, but the rising tide will soon make this unsafe. Climbing down the rusting iron rungs set into the wall, flirting with the idea of putting it back in the sea, if it will let me, my foot slips on the green slime and I'm brought up sharply. Once I'm beside it on the shingle, it is obvious the seal is just a baby, still showing some tufts of fluff from its birthing pelt. Exhausted and breathing badly, this youngster can't swim anywhere.

Small as it is, getting the slippery bundle up on to the pier is going to be a problem. Someone hands down a wooden fish box. The little seal is so small it will fit into one easily. We coax and roll it into the box with the judicious use of bits of wood and those thick, orange, fishermen's gloves. Having done this and feeling quite pleased with ourselves, we have a new problem. The seal's teeth, which are still quite active despite its tiredness, are right beside one of the handles we were going to use to lift the box. Solution number two: another fish box. Placing this on top and tying some carefully positioned rope, we have a perfect transport pod for our patient. A quick airlift up the harbour wall and we're done.

I brought the van down today instead of the car as it's big enough to take fairly sizeable animals. It's a Volkswagen Crew Bus. One of those square VWs, a bit like a brick aerodynamically, which can easily take the four boys and us parents. The middle bench seat can be unbolted and slid out if needed, so the van converts into a makeshift ambulance quite quickly. No need to do that today, though, now the transport pod is secure on the back shelf over the engine for warmth. I feel I should have brought my green flashing emergency light to complete the entertainment as we drive through the island to the hospital shed. Passing the school, small children's heads appear and rapidly disappear at the windows. How do they know what's going on?

Tipping the patient from the improvised transport pod to the hospital bed, I'm able to get a better look at it. Being this close to a wild seal should be exciting but the huge eyes are dull and lifeless, sad but still wary in this dark alien environment of rough straw and peering humans. Pity replaces excitement. Its pelt is covered in soft grey hairs and the thick bristly whiskers around its snout twitch with fear. Its snout is very moist, pouring mucus, what we used to call a 'snottery beak' when I was a kid at school. The compassion that I felt as a young boy, which insisted I become a doctor – returns unexpectedly, catching me off guard. I want to help.

Touching its body, there's a coldness, fish-like, the same as a severely shocked patient. Since it's not actually a fish (we won't need the police to deal with fishy business), we need to try to warm it up. I've rigged up a light above it with a 200-watt bulb as a temporary heat source. The little seal doesn't care what's going on as we wrap it up in an old blanket. It lies limply, coughing, sneezing, sad eyes far away searching for a lost mother. Expert advice is needed.

'Is that the seal rescue centre? Can I speak to Ben, please?'

'Speaking, what can I do for you?'

I explain who I am and what I've done so far.

'You're doing well, Doc, sorry we can't get out to you today, but we'll manage tomorrow I'm sure. The seal probably has seal "flu". It's a form of distemper virus that's killing hundreds of them. Have you taken its temperature?'

'How do I do that?'

I have visions of the little seal lying pathetically on the straw with a thermometer under its flipper.

'You need to take a rectal temperature.'

Okay, this is interesting. I need to stick a glass rod up a seal's ... bottom! I'm not sure I've even seen its bottom.

'Then you need to get lots of fluid into it; they get very dehydrated with mucus production.'

Now I'm starting to get worried. This isn't sounding straightforward at all.

'Have you got a nasogastric tube you can use? Perhaps one for calves?'

I suppress a laugh, imagining a patient's face if I pulled a calf feeding tube from my medical bag.

'I'll think of something. What liquid do I use to rehydrate?' I say, making myself behave professionally again.

'The best is herring broth. You need four or five herring made into a watery soup, perhaps with a little oatmeal. Then you feed around a pint and a half every four hours.'

Herring! I'm pretty sure there's none of them in stock in the dispensary.

'Anything other than herring soup?' I ask hopefully.

'You can use "Lectade" as well, although it's not so good. You know, the stuff they use for lambs and calves.'

If I ever have this life over again and I go to medical school, I must ask for a series of lectures on lambing and calving, possibly with some ornithology and sealology thrown in too. It's obvious my training was deficient in many ways. Why did I never have to rehydrate a seal when I worked in the east end of Glasgow?

'Okay, Ben, I'll see how I get on and I'll phone you if I'm stuck.' Still being professional.

'Great, Doc, you're doing a grand job. See you tomorrow.'

Time for the island to rally round. First, a phone call to the post office. Ann has an emergency supply of veterinary medicines we can use if we need. Next, a phone call to Ken to see about a calf feeding tube. I've helped him with his cattle before. Ken suggests a heat lamp, like they use for lambs. He doesn't have one but Billy at Seatter Farm might.

Returning to the little shed, armed with various implements, Maggie and I are ready to feed the sick seal pup. The heat lamp suspended above us is giving the whole place an eerie orangey-red glow, a bit like an intensive care unit at night. Outside, everything is silent, even the wind has stopped, hesitating before the storm arrives, waiting to see how things turn out. There's almost no life in the seal pup, lying on the straw bed as it concentrates solely on breathing, indifferent to the clatter of buckets, syringes and tubes as we prepare for our resuscitation attempt. As we approach, the huge eyes close and an exhausted sigh leaks from its nose as the little body slumps into the straw bed.

At least, there was little life in it until we tried to take its temperature! Carefully approaching the listless form from behind, I gently lift its tail. There's nothing to see, nowhere to place the thermometer grasped in my gloved right hand. Not a flinch or sound from the patient. Maggie positions the torch to let me see a little better.

'Is that where I should go?' An indentation appears in front of my hand.

This is as bad as putting a urinary catheter into an old woman on a foggy night, I think to myself.

Then I ask myself, *When did I ever try to catheterize someone on a foggy night?* I might be losing it now.

'Gently does it now, this feels right, slip the end of the thermometer in slowly ...'

'Whoa!' There are teeth, teeth everywhere. Apparently sticking a glass rod up a seal's bottom has amazing resuscitative properties. I jump back, instantly deciding to mark the animal's temperature down as 'cold' and leave it at that.

Next comes the feeding tube, which we have to get past those three rows of teeth and into its stomach. A bit like syphoning petrol from a tank, except we have a choice of tanks and it's vital we get the right tank. If the tube goes down into the lungs instead of the stomach, when we pour liquid in we will almost immediately kill our patient. It has enough liquid in its lungs from the flu.

Getting a decent hold on the patient before we can even try inserting the tube isn't proving easy. I don't know if you've ever noticed but there aren't handles on a seal. They only come with relatively small, slippery flippers that you can't hang on to. Paediatric know-how is needed. It wasn't unusual for a young child on the children's ward to refuse its antibiotics. Since the only alternative would be to put up a drip, it was occasionally necessary to wrap the child in a blanket and pop the medicine in, without the added issue of flailing arms and legs. Let's see how seals do when they're tightly wrapped in one of those packing blankets we saved from when we moved house.

There we are, a stroke of genius, a firmly held seal. The feeding tube slips down surprisingly readily, with almost nothing in the way of a fight. The pup must have tired itself out when we approached the blunt end earlier. Attaching the funnel, a tiny drop of Lectade is poured in to check the tube position. No chance of X-ray checks or testing an aspirate for acidity to let us know we're in the correct place, we have to rely on common sense. There's no increase in coughing or hint of sudden collapse so on we go with a pint of Lectade. The yellow liquid looks a bit like Lucozade without the fizz and probably isn't that different in make-up. We just have to wait and see if the patient responds now. Closing the door as quietly as we can, we let our patient rest in its little intensive care unit.

Outside, the arrival of the storm is apparent now. Something about the air before a storm hits warns you of its presence, a breath-holding, neurotic stillness surrounds you. Apprehension settles on the island, creeping along the shore, into the bays and over fields of stiff unflinching grass. The sea tugs anxiously at the skirt of the island, waves no longer lapping but grabbing the sand with tightly curled, urgent fists, slapping the rocks, hinting at turmoil further out. Birds recognize it too. Winter flocks of curlew fall silent and oystercatchers on the shore join them in the quiet. Silent and waiting.

At 4 a.m. there's a persistent beeping sound, an annoying descant piping, playing over a deep pulsing bass roar. The bed shudders slightly. Clawing myself awake, I realize the alarm is going off. The wind has picked up to a full gale and is blasting across the top of the chimney in the little bedroom next door. The chimney is only about twelve feet long and makes unearthly sounds in the wind. It's time to feed the young seal again. We managed feeds at 8 p.m. and midnight before we came to bed and another four hours have gone by. Both shivering as we try to dress in the half-light of the bedside lamp, we stumble round the room. Four o'clock in the morning is never a good time for a night call, even if it is just to the shed outside. Our body cortisol levels have fallen and all our impulses tell us we should be asleep. Nothing to be done but get on with it, though.

In the hospital shed, our patient is less than pleased to see us, snake-like hissing is coming from deep in the straw. Looking at each other, our eyes mirror the same question. Why are we standing half-dressed, dowsed in eerie orange light, in a vibrating, gale-blown shed while a seal hisses at us? Maggie raises her left eyebrow slightly, staring steadily at me and making her views quite clear!

We reach silent agreement that we're completely bonkers and carry on.

Another tube feed isn't on the list of things our patient wants to do. Recovering the ability to bend in the middle, the little seal presents the sharp end now, no matter what angle we approach from. Fortunately, it cannot climb out of its straw bed, as we had the foresight to put improvised cot sides up. Deciding discretion is the better part of valour, we escape as gracefully as we can, reversing into the gale, which derisively hurls rain at our bare legs. Laughing at the ludicrous escapade, we dive back through the door, getting thoroughly soaked in the process. Back at the duty station in the kitchen, the little black stove now glowing fiercely in the gale, we agree our patient is getting better and retire back to bed. Sleep comes eventually, while we listen to the comforting bass roar in the chimney and feel the slight shudder through the floorboards.

In the morning, the wind has gone. Checking on the seal at around 8 a.m., it seems just as lively as the night before and definitely not wanting to be fed. Ben, from the seal rescue centre, should be with us in an hour, so we box the seal again into its transport pod and go back to the harbour. There's about a three-hour window in the eye of the storm before the winds pick up again and we're stuck for another day. When we arrive, I decide to keep the seal inside the van to prevent it getting cold again.

We've been waiting for a good while now with no sign of Ben. I didn't realize he was coming in a RIB, an open inflatable dingy with a ridged bottom. These inshore craft can do the hour and a half journey from mainland in about twenty-five minutes given good sea conditions. As I hover on the harbour wall again the sea looks steely grey, calm as a millpond, but there's an unease in it, and a tangible apprehension in the air surrounding us. Weather patterns repeat as they have done for years. The clouds mimic the grey of the sea, but high above the island they appear to move faster than they should, an urgency in their movement as they are chased across the sky. Wavelets tug the shore again, always grasping, slapping down on the rocks once more. The little group of waiting fishermen, island men, is also quiet. Faces taut, restless eyes saying more than words can. There is risk in this gathering in, this seal rescue. Up until now it's simply been a bit of an unusual adventure, just a little bit of craziness. Last night's gale brought the danger into view. Fifteen miles of sea is a lot of water to get lost in and the currents are easily strong enough to take a small boat far out into the ocean.

Finally, a sigh of relief goes through the group, faces relax, becoming nonchalant with affirmations of barely convincing 'I told you so's'. Over an hour and a half late, the RIB appears round the headland, a cream and grey streak on the horizon slowly forming into the red-orange of the inflatable. Without hesitating, the tiny craft powers to the harbour steps to be held fast by the waiting hands. We've just over an hour before the wind picks up again.

Safely in the harbour, Ben tells us the engines stuttered and stalled just off Shapinsay, about a third of the way here. Both carburettors were stripped down and cleaned while they drifted at sea. Then they flew on before the gale, the two 40-horsepower outboards driving them forward once more. There's no more chatter, though, as the wind returns and puffs a warning through my hair. The seal is safely transferred in its pod, which is lashed to the seat, and inside ten minutes the RIB disappears at full speed round the headland again, out of sight. On its way to the seal sanctuary in Burray, gathered in to safety.

Hard Holding

I am Eid-ey,
The isthmus isle, the connector of tidal lands.

My birth hard won beneath the seas.
Corroded by desert winds; blown sands
driven into my faults,
I am
Flawed yet whole.
Formed by drawing all things to me
I hold them hard.

He will want to go now,
this man,
Go with his wife to the birthing of their child.
He shall not. He will wait.
Wait and Learn
Not all things are in his control.

9

Going

It seemed like a good idea when I said to Jenny we would hold an Easter egg rolling competition at Heatherlea. I hadn't really allowed for the lack of hills with suitable grassy slopes. It's not possible to roll your Easter egg in the heather. Ingenuity was required and, as I'm slowly learning, anything is possible on the island with a little lateral thinking. I've attached a length of plastic piping to the guttering above the upstairs bedroom window and this now slopes down to the corrugated roof of the porch. Another bucket and pulley system is in place to deliver the eggs to roof height before tipping them into the pipe to start their journey earthwards. Early tests have proved successful, after some minor adjustments.

Easter Sunday is freezing but at least the rain has stayed away. A gaggle of children have joined the geese in the garden, all with brightly decorated hard-boiled eggs of various types, including a goose egg. I once tried to eat a boiled goose egg for breakfast. It took twenty minutes to cook and once I'd finished eating it I didn't need any more food for the whole day. Anyway, I'm not sure the goose egg will fit down the pipe, we'll try it last.

Eggs rattle down the pipe then wobble across the corrugated roofing before wiping themselves out in the garden below. Any thoughts we may have had about eating our hard-boiled eggs afterwards are literally smashed. Slowly, the garden fills with egg shrapnel and a small crowd of seagulls is gathering along the ridge of the roof in anticipation. They have no chance of feasting yet, as the increasingly excited gaggle of little people is still in charge of the garden. Finally, it is time for the goose egg, which surprisingly does fit through the pipe, hurtling down on to the porch before flying up into the air to land with a dull thud on the grass below, completely unscathed. No wonder I didn't need anything else to eat that day, these things are solid. Having run out of ammunition for our Easter egg cascade, everyone charges into the kitchen for some hot soup and Easter cakes, leaving the gulls to their egg orgy.

Apart from the storm in January, our first winter has been gentle, with little of the relentless wild and unforgiving weather we had worried about. Work in the practice has been easy and gradually the little surgery, grubby and unloved at first, has been transformed into our homely workplace. The four boys love being here and have the freedom to roam where they like. The younger ones are eager to play in the walled garden all day if they can. Their childhood is now so much like my own. Open fires; paraffin lamps; Wellington boots; hills and heather. They do lack the little river I had running alongside the village green, dammed and fished perpetually throughout the summers. The beaches and seashore make up for this.

The medicine, the diagnoses and the cases are fascinating for such a small population. I had worried I would be bored and not have enough interesting work to keep my mind sharp. This isn't true – rarities are almost abundant here, for reasons I don't yet understand. Complex endocrine problems – cases where the hormone balance in the body is incorrect. Conditions that a doctor may expect to see only once in his life. The full spectrum of heart disease. The tiny practice regularly presents intriguing diagnostic puzzles that need to be carefully worked through. Each investigation and referral is carefully timed to the rhythm of the single boat and little plane that ferry people to Kirkwall. The drudgery of endless queues of irrelevance has gone. I'm more likely to be asked later than I would like about symptoms than presented with trivia.

Strangely, with all the true illnesses on the island, no one appears to consider they are unwell. They simply have complaints which need to be sorted to allow them to get on with life. Perhaps some of the newer arrivals are less resilient but they don't stay long, finding the testing of the island too intense. Moving south again to the familiar and predictable.

Two days after Easter, and Maggie has flown in to Kirkwall to see how our own little egg is coming on. She's now thirty-two weeks into her pregnancy and feeling really well. There are no signs of any problems, so we're beginning to put plans in place for June, when our fifth baby is due. Trevor is happy to come back as locum, especially as the weather should be fine then. Leaning on the fence behind the airport sheds while I wait for her, sheltered from a cutting north wind, I can just see the afternoon flight coming into view.

The plane banks and turns into the strengthening northerly as it completes its final approach. I can see Maggie in the rear window seat and wave to her as the plane shudders to a halt at the wooden huts. She climbs down from behind the wing and without lifting her head walks past me to the car. I reach out to take her hand but she pulls it away from me, hugging herself instead. Without a word, she opens the car door and sits down.

Looking straight ahead she says firmly, 'Take me home, now!'

'What happened?'

'Just take me home,' she says with her head down, obviously controlling the emotions churning inside her, which she wants no one else to see.

We drive in silence to the house and once in the kitchen allow the warmth of the black iron stove to drive out the bitter cold of the north wind. Only then does she cry, tears soaking my shirt as my arms hold her tight to me.

There is nothing to discuss, only plans to be made after today's maternity clinic visit in Kirkwall. Our baby is alive and well, but this could change at any time. Today's scan in the clinic shows the placenta lying low across the neck of the womb. Unless this moves upwards as the baby grows, then mother and baby could bleed to death during labour. Even the very act of growing, the stretching of the lower part of the womb that is inevitable at this stage of pregnancy, could peel the placenta away and bleeding will follow. A sea of blood separating the baby from its mother. If labour starts before this movement takes place, then the only course of action is immediate caesarian section. This is not something the island – I – can do. Maggie must fly to Aberdeen and stay there, remote, for the next six weeks.

Multiple phone calls are made through the evening. The boys all spoken to. Normality maintained. But not for Maggie and me. We've never been separated for more than a few days, we're used to being together, even at work. The long night lies before us, while the wind, steady as a flowing river, drags cold air down from the north, depositing it on the island and in the seas beyond. The room is cold as we lie side by side, fingertips touching to maintain connection, all too aware again of the unpredictability, the fragility of life. Suddenly too fragile for us to hold each other in case we cause the baby harm. A real but illogical fear. Three weeks ago, Maggie was dressed in baby-bump-stretched orange oilskin trousers, ready to sail to the tiny island of Auskerry in an open boat if necessary. There was a baby due there too. She had gone alone, to cover Stronsay, our neighbouring island where the doctor had become seriously unwell. He was flown direct from the island to Aberdeen. Tonight she waits for her flight.

Morning comes, and we keep the routine the same. School bags are packed and lunches crammed into boxes.

'Say goodbye to Mummy and give her big hugs, guys, she'll be away a little while until we get the new baby,' and, 'Yes, we'll send her lots of pictures and you can write letters.'

'See you soon, Mummy!'

'Bye, Mummy!'

That word 'bye', said lightly but sounding short, nerve-racking, final. The island isolation is increasing the sense of a last 'goodbye'. It doesn't help, her being a doctor and knowing too much. Maggie has seen the effects of antepartum haemorrhage, the sudden catastrophic bleeding that comes out of the blue in later pregnancy. She has anaesthetized women, white as ghosts, lying with their head tilted down to the floor, keeping the blood flowing to their brain, and reducing the blood spilled on the floor. A 'crash section'. The only way to save baby and mother.

'Goodbye, boys, be good for Daddy and I'll be back before you know it.' Her mother's voice, steady and even, as she smiles and waves them into the school Land Rover.

Claire arrives to watch Michael and Murray, while we drive to the airstrip. A bag filled with the essentials for waiting – nightgowns, toiletries, crochet needle and wool, cross-stitch – is laid in the back of the car. Hidden underneath these essentials for survival is a little optimism. A white baby jacket with pearlized buttons alongside a satin-ribbon-trimmed bonnet and a pair of tiny bootees. Part of the growing collection prepared through the winter, always in white, as we never want to know the baby's sex before the birth. A smile crossed my face as the baby clothes went into the bag, remembering my early knitting efforts for Martin, our first son. A pair of button-under dungarees, again in white, knitted through the long night duties on the paediatric ward.

At the airstrip we stay in the car instead of facing folks in the hut. The wind is still strong, while a clear blue sky hides behind piles of black thunder clouds, rolling south. Silence returns once more as the plane comes into sight, buffeted and shaken by the wind as it turns to land. We kiss briefly in the car and then, pushing the door into the gale, step out slowly. Holding hands, a finger grip, light but constant, we grasp on to each other as we cross to the plane. Without turning, Maggie climbs behind the wing once more and into the plane. Placing the 'waiting' bag into the hold, I turn away too.

The twin-engined Islander taxis away to the south and spins slowly into the headwind. The gusts of wind, driving across the island from the north, carry the engines' roar away to the south. The only sound is the wind, hissing through the coarse, brittle grasses, the whining in the power lines down on the shore, and the plaintive cry of a single curlew. As the plane's front wheel lifts from the runway there's a furious crash of thunder and the island skies hurl a deluge of hail and sleet at the struggling white shape, making it hesitate for a moment before fighting its way into the sky. The island's irrational fury is tangible, as if it never wants anyone to leave. Maggie is out of sight. My eyes follow the straight line of the lichen-grey fence posts to the horizon, but I can't make the line connect with the plane in the sky. There's an emptiness deep inside me, and the first tendrils of fear creep into the hollow. The harsh, hissing sounds of the winds in the grasses stay with me, inside my head, as if I'm being laughed at. I walk back to the car and go home.

So now we must wait too. Driving over the hill from the airstrip and down to Heatherlea, the house looks dismal. Lichen-encrusted flaking grey paint on the old house competes with the new harled surgery box stuck on the end of the building. A box that nearly had the lid prised off in the winter storm. Not a house to come home to after the birth of a child. Anger forces its way into the emptiness to replace the creeping edge of fear. Time to fill the waiting with physical tasks to use up my energy and still my thoughts.

Back at the house, opening the kitchen door, my time is soon taken up with the younger boys. The youngest, now affectionately known as 'Peedie Breeks' or 'Peedie' for short, will soon be two years old and is very vocal. 'Peedie' is Orcadian for little or small and can be applied to people and objects alike. Our 'Peedie' may be small in stature but not in temperament. He has instantly replaced Mum with Dad and when Claire tries to do anything with him he responds with, 'Daddy do it,' and folds his arms defiantly, scowling under his white fringe of hair.

'Come here, pal, what's the problem?'

'My hor'sh.'

'Oh, I see,' I say, looking at the red and cream wheelie horse sitting in the middle of the room. 'And what's the problem with it, then?'

'It'sh arsing about!' and he wriggles down from my arms to storm out of the room.

There must be a way to be Dad and Doctor. There's no choice but to be both; to be all three really, to be Mum too. I can't stop being the doctor and any thoughts of leaving to be with Maggie quickly disappear as Trevor, my locum, isn't available yet. Anyway, my leave must be kept for the birth when it comes. *If it comes!* The thought steals its way in and sits waiting for me to notice it.

The next morning, after a disorganized first day, Martin and Matthew are sent off to school and I attempt to straighten the day out in my mind. I can't. I'm still brooding on the call to Maggie last night. Safely in the antenatal ward in Aberdeen, she's uneasily battening down for the long wait. We know nobody down there, all our friends are in the west of Scotland. Paradoxically, the isolation seems greater for her now she's away from the island in an alien environment. Doctors don't become patients easily; we are disorientated, like looking in a mirror with everything the wrong way around. We're used to moving freely, wandering into duty rooms, getting answers to our questions or finding them for ourselves in records and reports. As patients we're disabled, unsure of the language to use. Should we use our technical language or the language of a patient? In our confusion, we often choose to say very little, closing in on ourselves and letting events unfold. Aware of her confusion and anxiety, I couldn't find the words to help her, and uneasiness settled on us both when the hesitant call finished.

After two days of coping, juggling work and home with varying degrees of success, Nana, Maggie's mum, has arrived, having thoroughly enjoyed the second flight from Kirkwall. The weather was benign, with late spring sunshine and gentle winds. Her views of the approaching island were spectacular as the plane dropped down to the tiny green airstrip. The island welcomed her, drawing her in carefully. The house, however, was not so welcoming, glowering at her as we came over the hill from the airport. It's time to channel some of that anger, to straighten out my disorientation and do some practical work.

After the chaos of the daytime, a little evening routine is forming. With tea finished and washed up, the older two boys sit down and we tackle homework together. Nana baths Peedie Breeks in the kitchen sink, despite his protests.

'Daddy do it!'

'No, Daddy's busy, come and play with your duck.'

'I'sh hate my duck.'

'Don't be silly, it's a nice duck. Come and give it a bath, it's got a dirty face.'

'I'sh want my hor'sh, it's dirty too.'

'It's too big for the sink. There, now, in you go,' and, 'Will you sit down, you'll fall.'

'I'sh looking at ducks out the window.'

We shut the splashing protests out by closing the living-room door.

Mikey, although not at school yet, joins in with his homework, which he demands each night. Sitting in the corner by the window, he practises his writing and drawing for Mum. He seems unperturbed that she's away, although he did punch me in the stomach today after I teased him and said Mum was rubbish. Matthew is sitting close to me on the couch, cuddled in, as we do some maths homework. He likes a cuddle. Before Mum went away he was already struggling with his reading – we're beginning to wonder if he may be dyslexic like my sister. Mum going away suddenly has added to his upset; school isn't his favourite place at the moment. Martin is sitting in Mum's seat by the fire, working away on his own. It's difficult to know what Martin thinks; he keeps lots of things to himself.

With the chores and homework done, there is time to play. A gentle drizzle has started tonight, though, blowing mist, drenching the garden, smurring the living-room windows. Playing outside isn't an option. The gang has decided we should play Cowboys and Indians, and multiple ambushes are creating havoc through the Badlands of Heatherlea. Whispering and screaming alternate as, throughout the wild country, gunfire cracks from high-plains bedrooms and the desert dining room, and echoes across stairwell cliff. I am the sole Indian, mounting various attacks on Cowboys hidden in canyons, in cupboards and gulches under beds. The most daring attack yet is made up stairwell cliff.

Dust bunnies spin down the stairs as the cowboys gallop up the steep slope of Stairway Rise to gain the heights of the

Heatherlea Badlands. The little posse quickly disappears into Bedroom Gulch, the youngest – Peedie-Breeks McGraw – clutching his faithful Pingu (an incongruous black and white penguin knitted by Maggie) in one hand and his six-shooter in the other. Regrouping in Bedroom Gulch they start to make plans. Marty the Brain, Matt the Bite, Mikey the Redhead and Peedie-Breeks McGraw.

'List'n, watch out for him,' says Marty the Brain, the oldest of the group.

'He came in the window the last time.' Matt the Bite looks round anxiously.

'I'sh he there now?' A small white-headed Peedie dives to the door.

'No, Peedie, don't look out, we're not ready!'

'Where is he?'

'It's too quiet.'

'If he comes along the landing, we'll see him first, we can jump him!'

'C'n I'sh jump from the top bunk?'

'No, Peedie, you'll hurt yourself. Get under the bed, quickly!'

'Shhhh, I heard something!' says Mikey the Redhead, still suspicious from an encounter with me in the afternoon when I said Mum was rubbish.

The only sound is running water, far away in the kitchen, splashing in the sink. Then a single creak of a stair.

Then nothing.

Unknown to the waiting cowboys, Big Chief Sitting Dad has climbed the outside of Stairwell Cliff. Stepping on Telephone Seat Rock, he's swung across Landing Gap and is hidden from view just over Banister Ridge. Clinging on by his fingernails, he's ready to spring in front of the little posse. For now, though, he waits, considering his final attack (and the drop down the stairwell if he slips ...).

Whispering, low, urgent.

'Why does he always wait before he attacks?' Matt the Bite is still anxious.

'Don't trust him,' hisses Mikey the Redhead. 'He said Mum was a rubbish mum today.'

'He was joking, Mikey, he's always joking.' Age gives Marty the advantage on the topic.

'I punched him in the stomach!'

'Why'd you do that?'

'Dunno when he's joking, his face was serious.'

'Shhhh, be quiet, we can't hear him coming!'

'Shove over, Martin, m'leg's sticking out the bed.' The Bite is getting more nervous by the minute.

'We should've split up an' ambushed him from the bathroom!' Mikey, still on the attack.

'Nah, there's nowhere to hide.'

'Why's he taking so long?'

'We'll have to go and see.'

'I'sh can go!'

'Peedie, stay here! Come back!'

'I'sh need a pee!'

'Shhh ... Listen, I heard the stair creak.'

'We'll have to go and see,' says Marty the Brain. 'Peedie is desperate now!'

'You look out, Marty.'

'Can you see anyth—'

'Aaahhhhh!' Screaming cowboys dart everywhere. 'Run, Peedie, run to the bathroom!'

'Where was he?'

'Keep running,' pants Marty the Brain. 'He climbed up the outside of the stair.'

'He's crazy!' cries Matt the Bite.

'I told you, don't trust him!' storms Mikey the Redhead.

It may take a little longer for the pardners to settle tonight.

Finally, around 7.30 p.m., there's time for myself. Making myself comfortable on telephone seat 'rock' at the foot of the stairs, I'm ready for a good chat with Maggie. You have to call the ward staff first and they bring Maggie to the phone in the little room beside the duty room. Except, tonight she's not allowed to come to the phone. The clerk asks me to wait while they take the patient trolley phone to her bedside. The emptiness deep inside returns, forcing me to make myself stay calm.

My hands are shaking as the phone goes back into its cradle; I need to sit quietly for a while. Without warning, my world turns chaotically upside down. All she did was go to the toilet and when she stood up blood poured down her legs on to the floor. Not a few drips in the water of the toilet pan, which looks like pints, but actual pints, spreading slowly on the tiled floor. She hit the alarm button and stood there shivering with fright and cold as her blood pressure fell. She expected to be in theatre in minutes, one of those crash sections she had seen so many of. Instead, a bucket and mop unceremoniously wiped her blood away, then she was mopped and put to bed.

I want to scream out, to shout, to cry, but I can't, I never can. Even as a child I would think about things before reacting. I would draw things together, facts, feelings, sounds, connecting them and laying them out in a line, then planning a way forward. Days would stretch out in front of me like a line into the future as I watched for problems ahead. Sometimes the line is long, spanning years, sometimes short, the connections made rapidly. Perhaps I should act like a normal husband and ask myriad questions, demand answers. I don't. I can't. It's not how my brain works. Baby's heart rate is stable and showing no signs of upset from the bleed. There is nothing more to be done just now. Nothing is in my control, Maggie has to rest, and we have to wait.

Emotionally, I'm a wreck, sitting alone beside the dying embers of the peat fire. Knowing the right answer and living with it are two very different things. I need to be able to see the way forward, to connect the various elements of a situation, to line them up and examine them to find pathways through. These rapidly planned routes and actions allow me to appear calm, in control. People have said to me how flexible I am, laid-back, they think. I'm not, I just think quickly and reach solutions, joining the dots with straight lines that appear curved and flowing. Antoni Gaudi once said, 'The straight line is made by man, the curved line by God.' In disorder, when my lines are forcibly bent, like now, I need God to sort them out. Not the universe-creating God, aloof and distant from us, or some stone edifice in a church building, some mythical creature of chariots and pillars of smoke, but someone who will talk to me readily, openly, disagree with me and challenge me.

The emptiness inside me is now filled with fear. Fear of losing Maggie to a further catastrophic bleed. I have to pray. Not Sunday-school-gentle-Jesus praying – this is a raw, urgent, tantrum of prayer. A cry driven by the unfairness of being disabled by the island, the injustice of being unable to hold Maggie and lessen her fear of losing the baby. I don't ask for anything in this foot-stamping tirade, I demand it. Demand God doesn't let Maggie die. I don't threaten anything, to stop believing or stop caring, my inner voice simply shouts, instructs God in what he has to do. My mind is irrationally furious with him for a long time – how dare he stop me holding Maggie, how dare he take her from me. On and on and on until I am no longer in control. Only then, gradually, to begin with almost imperceptibly, at the height of my tirade, the words come. Not in my head but around me. Not spoken but there in my consciousness, even as my rage continues. They form and take shape, as the rain on the windows clears and the island sunlight bleeds into the room.

'Be still and know that I am God.' It's then I cry.

There are no more signs of bleeding when I call the ward again. Maggie, asleep now in a private room beside the nurses' station, has pads on, which are checked every hour for more bleeding. She'll have a long night. Exhaustion takes over, and after packing the stove in the kitchen with coal, turning the spinners tight shut to get a slow burn, I make my way to bed. Martin and Michael are sound asleep in their bunk beds. Martin wrapped in a twisted duvet like a snail, holding things to himself even as he sleeps. Michael in a coma, flat on his back. Peedie and Matthew are asleep in the room next to me. A tiny snow-white head lying beside his black and white penguin. Pulling the fireguard tight across their little coal fire, its embers still glowing red, I allow myself to go through to bed and fall immediately into an unsettled sleep.

The sound of screaming wakes me. Stumbling and falling in the half-light, I go through to the next room. The faint red glow from the dying fire bathes Matthew's distraught face as he sits bolt upright on his top bunk, eyes wide open. He's not awake though. His night terrors are getting worse. Dreams of imagined danger deep in his subconscious. Holding him, rocking him gently, we stay locked together until he falls properly asleep again. I'm grateful to hold someone tonight and make their fear go away.

10

Why?

It's two weeks since Maggie flew to Aberdeen and fog has settled today, shrouding everything in a clinging dampness that seeps into every crack and crevice. The wind still blows. Nothing is clear, as the clawing wetness crawls inside me. I need bright windswept days. There is no light today. Thick suffocating cloud obliterates the sun, an oppressive mud-like gloom sitting on everything, sucking energy from me and dulling my ability to think. I feel as though I'm drowning in a thin sea. I could swim if the water held me up but it doesn't, and slowly I slide down and down. I keep brooding over the reasons we came so ridiculously far north, why we are where we are, why I placed Maggie in danger. I was sure we were in the wrong place a year ago, stuck in the mundane, drowning in the perceived irrelevance of suburban Glasgow. I'm not sure we're in the right place now.

To uproot my whole family from the comfort and ease of an urban lifestyle to a house with no soul, damp, dispirited, overrun with mice, where the carpets lift from the floor with every gust of wind. Wind which paradoxically blows any vestige of heat into the sea while sucking the front door firmly shut in the slightest gale. A grey glowering place, sitting in the middle of a wind-riven peat bog. Why did we move here, to this place where wind and weather dictate? A thin, anaemic land of rock and sandstone and bog where the harsh countryside only reluctantly allows us to live.

Why? Why? Why had I been so restless? Others looking at me thought I was happily married. I had four sons, a beautiful house and a promising suburban practice that might soon be mine exclusively, if my partners' promises were to be believed. But a nagging sense of dissatisfaction – a little knotweed of a thought – kept digging away at me, disrupting the subsoil of my life. The roots of this dissatisfaction were breaking through the foundations of my marriage. Annoyance, no, inexpressible anger at my partners in the practice was bottled up inside me and only overflowed at home. My sudden outbursts at minor injustices and perpetual prickliness of mood wore Maggie down as she tried to cope with her work and family life. We hadn't been talking openly to each other for a while. Facing the opposite way in bed, avoiding the contentious issue of my behaviour.

The boys weren't exempt from my moods either. One day I would happily play football in the back garden or have mock battles with Super Soaker water guns. The next, I could be roaring inappropriately at some minor misdemeanour. Like the time Matthew accidentally smashed a plant pot into a thousand pieces, sending pottery and soil cascading down the stairs. Suddenly I was incandescently angry. So much so that he ran and hid beneath our bed until rescued by Maggie, whose quiet she-wolf rage quelled mine instantly, leaving me alone and ashamed at my anger. Anger that should have been aimed directly at the cause, had I been able to see it. My relentless unhappiness, hidden beneath a facade, a pleasant outward veneer, was stretching the bond between Maggie and me. The bond that allowed us to work seamlessly, lovingly, professionally in the past, was being eroded to breaking point.

Work was grinding me down. Only the excitement of the really unusual was strong enough to pique my interest. The day I stopped at a road traffic accident on my morning rounds was one of the times when there was a real sense of fulfilment. When I was doing what I was trained to do, making the technicalities of care exciting again. A man, an urban tramp (as we knew them then), had been struck by a car crossing the road in the pouring rain and was lying drenched on the tarmac. His lips were blue-black, blood seeping from the wound at the back of his head. The car that had struck him was stationary now, sitting at a crazy angle to the road, one wheel up on the pavement, the engine still running. Another car pulled up in front was protectively corralling the old man, who lay motionless on the road, his stained overcoat scrunched up beneath him, making his back arch, positioning him in a permanent seizure. He was dying.

I spent the next hour kneeling beside him on the road while a stain of urine spread from under him. Focussed only on the technical, never considering the person I was treating, I concentrated solely on restarting his breathing and was triumphant when finally I managed it. Eventually he was lifted into the ambulance with a spinal board and neck brace in place, his pink face covered with an oxygen mask while a crew member looked after his airway. As they did, a blink of sunshine broke through the clouds and sparked briefly off a single gold earring he was wearing. Looking back now, it seems incongruous somehow, that earring. Why was it there? What did it mean about who he was, who he had been? These questions would need answers now, but back then I didn't waste time on them. I had done my job. He may not survive the massive head injury he'd suffered but he had been given a chance and that's all I was meant to do. I turned away to tell the very wet young policewoman who was waiting for my statement that I would see her in the surgery in the afternoon. I needed a change of clothing and the accident had delayed my morning's home visits.

Not that the visits couldn't wait. They were just another series of similarity. Illness driven by self-neglect – mostly smoking and alcohol. The people were nice enough when you called on them but there was nothing to really get my teeth into. More inhalers for asthmatics, antibiotics for bronchitis, anti-inflammatories for arthritics and inevitable snotty-nosed children who should have come to surgery (Mummy thought they shouldn't go out in the cold air), while Granny sits in the corner of the room, coughing.

It was only four years since I started in general practice and already the patterns of each day were becoming chronic, repetitive. The initial excitement of working independently, making my own diagnoses, writing my own prescriptions, had worn off and I was worn down by the sameness of daily routine. The only real variation was in the quantity of similarity; variety was rare. Oh, the people were different enough, pleasant to talk to, but I didn't train for nine years to talk to people. I put all that effort in to make a difference treating illness, curing disease so that people can get on with their lives.

Finally managing to finish the morning round of home visits and grab a quick lunch, I made it back to the surgery just in time for my afternoon patients. The young policewoman was standing, waiting. They never sit down, the police, always stand, reinforcing their position with their posture. In among gathering other details, she stopped the official questioning and wanted to know how the rough sleeper was. I directed her to the hospital. Delayed again, I eventually started seeing my patients.

'Come in. Nice to see you again. Come and have a seat.'

Not an act on my part. I did like seeing people and talking to them. I just didn't understand why I didn't seem to be making a difference. The illnesses persisted. Sometimes they changed form but they persisted. I couldn't really make them go away. Not like being in hospital, where we saved a life, prevented a cardiac arrest from killing the patient or removed a septic appendix from the fevered child. That work was done by specialists treating narrow bands of disease. I had hoped in general practice there would be a broad range of different illnesses to treat, diagnoses to explore. There wasn't, and even when there was a hint of an interesting case, I would have to refer it to the specialists I was trying to avoid becoming.

I made it as far as the third patient on my afternoon schedule when I was faced with an angry father. The feeling of satisfaction I felt when I managed to get the urine-soaked man breathing again, both of us lying in pools of rainwater and blood, trickled away. Slowly, it dissolved in the banality of afternoon surgery, invalidating two hours spent on the rain-soaked roadside. The father had brought his son to see me without an appointment and despite saying I would fit him in when I could, he refused to wait and burst into my surgery. After carefully examining the young boy and finding nothing much wrong with him, I quietly asked the youngster to sit outside the room. Closing the door gently, I allowed the growing frustration I felt to explode. I grabbed his father by the lapels and pinned him to the door. I didn't care what his reasons were for bursting in like that, I just wanted him to know how I felt.

The slow choking-out of satisfaction was unsettling me like the insidious roots of knotweed which eat at the foundations of buildings. Why did it germinate and take root? Was it when one of my senior partners, due to retire soon I hoped, came to the door of our house and berated Maggie when I was out because he couldn't find me? Perhaps, but that was a recurring issue which would pass, as they always did. The first time I was forced to consider what was happening, when a sense of being in the wrong place encroached on me, came on 21 December 1988.

Most evenings in winter we sat in the comfortable back sitting room, watching television while the boys played above us in the upstairs playroom. Their excitement at the approach of Christmas was already heightened by my staging of the theft of their old bikes by Santa's elves. Tiny bells rang in the night and doors mysteriously opened and closed as our children, dripping with interrupted sleep, listened from the landing above.

In the morning their bikes were gone. We couldn't afford to buy new ones, so I'd been stripping and repainting the old ones in secret ever since. At five to eight that night the TV programme was interrupted by a newsflash that was both unbelievable and real at the same time. Pan AM Flight 103 had been blown from the sky over Lockerbie.

As we listened to the report, the horror mingled with a sense of needing to help. I kept all my equipment in the car after the pedestrian accident, when I had had nothing with me, and I was only an hour away from the aeroplane crash site by motorway. Continuing to listen to the details, though, it became very clear that there would be no one alive to help. We sat in silence, hearing only the sounds of the planes taking off and landing at the nearby airport, as slowly the realization set in. We were under the flight path of Flight 103, one of the many high-flying planes that crossed the sky above us. Travelling as fast as it does, the plane could have been above us eight minutes later. The children playing above Maggie and me, the dog at my feet, all of us were nearly in the wrong place at the wrong time.

To try to combat the sameness of daily practice I'd learned a new skill – hypnotherapy. I thought perhaps I could make a difference with a new approach to problems. Actually, I found I was quite good at it and had built up a minor reputation in the area. So much so that a lady who was not my patient came to see if I could help her with an anxiety issue. My usual practice was to have an initial assessment session to see if the technique might work, then to start therapy sessions. The lady had been in a minor road traffic accident and ever since then she had been unable to get into a car, paralysed by the fear that the incident was just a precursor to a major event.

'Come and lie down over here on the couch and we'll see how we get on.'

'No.'

'Why not?'

'I can't lie down. It's like dying.'

'Okay ... we can do this while you sit up. Make yourself more comfortable in the chair and we'll get started. Are you comfortable now?'

'Yes. I'm fine here.'

'Good, now listen quietly, carefully to my voice,' I said, as I gradually modulated my speech to her breathing pattern. 'Listen to my voice, slowing your breathing, all the time listening to my voice.'

As I went through my routine I gradually relaxed myself as well, marrying my rhythms to the patient's. My voice quietened and deepened as we established connection – control, I suppose.

'Now your eyelids begin to feel heavy, sleepy. Let your eyes become heavier and heavier, heavier and heavier with each breath until they gently close. Heavier and heavier ...'

'No!' she said, immediately alert and awake. 'I can't do that. I'm sorry, I just can't!'

I'd had people who couldn't relax, settle themselves enough to undergo therapy but I'd never had someone who couldn't shut their eyes at all for me. She was apologetic and distraught at the same time, desperately wanting help. I had no choice but to carry on the session with her eyes wide open even though I'd never seen hypnosis done that way. It was a bizarre, disconcerting session where I took her back into an imaginary car, carefully closing the door, while all the time she sat looking straight at me. No flickers of eyelids, tightening of the corner of her mouth, quickening in breathing. Nothing to suggest she was upset by the thoughts she couldn't even talk about in the pre-therapy session. I was in complete control of this lady's state of mind while she sat there looking at me. Once the session was complete I woke her up, as it were, suggesting we meet up in a week and plan the next steps.

Before the end of the week I had a phone call from her.

'I'm fine, Doctor. Completely better.'

'Really? How did that happen, what happened?'

'Well, when I left your surgery I felt really well, so I went to the phone box and called my husband. When he arrived, I opened the car door and got in. We drove home ...'

I did it. I was able to completely cure someone at last.

Control their anxiety and, through the simple use of words and sounds, let them get on with life. Amazing. My next hypnotherapy patient was due that afternoon and I couldn't wait.

'Come in. What can I help you with today?'

'I want to stop smoking.'

'Excellent. Before we start, I want you to do a little test for me,' I said, suppressing the look of disappointment on my face before it surfaced.

'Give me a cigarette, please.'

'Do you smoke?' he asked, as he handed me it.

I crushed it between my fingers and threw it in the bin, all the while watching his face tighten and his breathing quicken ever so slightly.

'Now you take one and do the same, please.'

'I can't,' he said, with a defeated look in his eyes.

'And I'm sorry but my experience is that until you can crush that cigarette, we won't succeed. You may stop briefly but you'll start again.'

Smoking and alcohol. Again and again. Maybe I should have tried to help but what was the point?

Morning surgeries continued in their prescribed pattern. A never-ending stream of similarity queued each morning to see me. The first come, first served surgery schedule gathered twenty to thirty people in a silent room, all waiting to come into the consulting room that perched on the edge of the pavement – a converted shop front with a large frosted glass window to obscure the view. I could hear the conversation of the people in the street as I sat there. One morning, just as I was seeing sick-line number three, there was a scream of rubber on the road outside and an almighty slam of metal into metal, followed by that silence in which the world takes stock of what's happened. The receptionist burst through the door.

'Get outside now, there's been a terrible accident.'

'What happened ...?'

'It looks like an old man has pulled his car out in front of a lorry full of sand.'

I looked out the door and then dived back in.

'Call police and ambulance.'

'Already done ... Go!'

The street was quiet, shocked into silence by the insult to its natural rhythm. A freeze-frame of stationary people rooted in time. An old man, turning to see what had happened, with a brown trilby hat in his hand; a mother with a pushchair, frozen, with one wheel half off the pavement; a lady in a red coat, her hand at the pillar box, refusing to let go of the envelope. In front of me was the vacant space the car had pulled out of and the car itself, spun around and facing back to the place it wished it had never left. The bonnet was mangled, crumpled like a discarded piece of paper. The windscreen non-existent.

Through the shattered frame I could see a man suspended by his seatbelt, slumped forward in the driver's seat with his head hanging down.

Finally, I got my legs to move, breaking myself free from the scene. When I reached the mangled side of the car, the dashboard was still bright with red and orange lights. Somehow the hazard warning lights had come on in a vain attempt to prevent disaster. Carefully, I reached through the smashed side window and switched off the engine. The smell of rubber still clung to the air but there was no smell of fuel. Inside, the man was beginning to snore, long, struggling ineffective attempts to suck air into his lungs. His face was livid.

I pulled hopelessly at the driver's door, which was bent beyond use, and gave up. With one hand I held his chin up and immediately there was a long, gurgling intake of air into his starving lungs. My other hand searched for a pulse in his neck, which was gratifyingly strong. What now? It was only then I realized that my stethoscope was still draped around my shoulders. Quickly, with my free hand I shoved the end of my tubes into his shirt and listened. Both lungs seemed to be filling with air and his heart was strong at that moment. I ran my hand down on to his stomach and sides. He didn't seem to mind that, there was no wincing or grimacing.

'Hello, hello – can you hear me?' I said, shaking him a little with my free hand.

Nothing. He was deeply unconscious, probably from smashing his head on the doorpost beside him when the lorry slammed into him.

'I'm going to stay with you until we can get you out,' I continued. He might still have been able to hear me even if he couldn't respond.

Why was there no ambulance yet? How long had it been? A quick look at my watch told me why – 9.41 a.m. – it had only been two minutes since I left the surgery. I might have stepped out of the freeze-frame but I was still in slow motion. I needed to keep his airway open, but I couldn't do it from here; reaching through the window wasn't working so I let his head fall gently forward and he immediately stopped breathing. Giving the rear passenger door no option, I yanked at its handle, forcing the hinges, and clambered into the back seat. Reaching round the headrest, I gripped each side of his head and pulled slowly upwards until thankfully he started breathing again. Then I waited.

Outside the car, there was a developing fuss of police. Blue lights flashed, reflecting from shop windows. Ambulancemen arrived with bags of equipment. Oxygen was placed on the man's face, an airway attempted and rejected. All the while I was fixed in place, the one thing keeping the man alive at present. He was trapped in the front seat, his feet caught beneath the pedals, with no way of extricating him. I waited in my bubble of inactivity while the outside world was full of people organizing, shifting, measuring. Inside, there was just me and the man – breathing.

Slowly, I regulated my breathing, relaxing my shoulders with each breath, hypnotizing myself to reduce the developing ache in my arms, mentally shutting out the intrusive activity to concentrate solely on keeping the man alive. The smell of burned rubber persisted, invading the bubble surrounding me. The noise outside, the frenetic activity wasn't allowed in my hypnotic cocoon, I shut it out. But the smell had crept in. A fragment of the moment when the world stopped, and a man was offered the chance to die. The man whose life I literally held in my hands now.

The bubble burst when the ambulancemen offered to take over and give me a rest but I was concerned the man might have injured his neck as well as his head, so I stayed here. A neck brace was slipped into place, so the weight was reduced now. Heads are surprisingly heavy.

'We're going to have to cut him out, Doc,' said a voice from the fire crew, who had arrived now too. 'It'll be a bit noisy briefly. You okay with that?'

'Yep.'

'We'll put this helmet on then and these goggles. Don't look at the windows or cutters when we tell you.'

'Okay, you carry on.'

The rear windscreen was carefully removed, its rubber sealing strip peeled off and the glass lifted clear. The nearside passenger doors were opened wide until the only things between me and the outside world were six metal posts holding the roof up. The skin of my bubble was well and truly broken now.

'Look down now, Doc.'

Huge hydraulic cutters gripped the first doorpost and sliced it in half as easily as tin snips on kitchen foil. In what seemed like seconds the entire roof was lifted away. I was left kneeling in the open air in the back of a convertible, watched by a growing crowd of bystanders. The rest of the extrication moved at speed as the man was freed from his trap and laid gently on a spinal board. My hands were prised from the side of his head as the ambulanceman controlled his patient's neck from now on.

Quite suddenly, I was redundant. No one seemed to care what I did as the various emergency crews went about their business. The ambulance siren sounded as the vehicle sped away down the street. The sound stretched and slowed, then vanished. Turning through 360 degrees, reviewing the whole scene, I felt displaced. Anger flickered deep inside me as I looked at the onlookers, the voyeurs. Why had they intruded into my bubble? Turning again before the anger flared, I crossed the pavement towards the surgery door, adjusting my stethoscope on my shoulders as I went. Pushing open the door, I saw the hands of the old Bakelite wall clock sitting at 11.17 a.m. An hour and three quarters since I left. Brushing off the fragments of rubber and seat stuffing sticking to my trousers, I looked round the waiting room. Two old ladies were waiting. Sitting with their hands folded on their laps and pleasant, welcoming smiles, beaming at me. 'We knew you were busy, Doctor, but don't worry, we don't mind waiting.' I quickly opened the reception-room door and went in.

'What are they still doing here?'

'They stayed. When everyone else said they could come back later, they stayed, I'm afraid. Said it was important they see you. Are you okay?'

'Why?'

'We were worried about you ... all that noise of cutting.'

'No, why have they stayed?'

'I think they have colds ...'

As I slammed the consulting room door behind me I could just hear the receptionist say, 'Dr MacKay says he's left you the two house calls. He has a golf match this afternoon ...'

In the midst of all this turmoil there was one place where I could forget. Shut out all the nonsense around me. Nonsense which, if I'm truthful, was as much about my attitude as anything. That evening was choir rehearsal night and we'd gathered in the upper hall for our weekly practice. This was an invitation-only choir, voices selected by the conductor to match his requirements. I loved it. There, I didn't have to think. I was not in charge of anything. There was only one item I must attend to and that was the note I must sing. Everything else was decided for me: practice timing – 7.30 p.m. – not 7.31 p.m.; choice of music – the conductor's; phrasing of lyrics – the conductor's; dynamics of the piece – the conductor's; tea break – 8.30 p.m. Everything was out of my control except the sound I made. I literally had one job – to sing. Concentration is important, as I naturally sing slightly flat, and I'm grateful for that. If my voice was perfect, then singing would become easy and my mind could have wandered off, back to the events of the day. Breathing, phrasing, singing the note from top down instead of scooping up to it. The effort didn't just block out the day, it obliterated it. Only making music existed, blending my voice with those around me until I sank into anonymity and peace.

At Christmas we gathered for drinks and a buffet at the conductor's house. Each of us received a Christmas card, inside which was our report for the past year. Always a compliment followed by an area for improvement. That year, mine said: 'Your tone has improved greatly and your contribution to the bass line is solid.' There was always a but though. 'Be more confident and sing out. Consider taking a solo next session.' Being a solid bass is good, no one wants freelancing on the bass line, we leave that to the sopranos. I wasn't sure about the solo though. I didn't feel confident enough to be solely responsible for a song. Everyone else relying on me alone.

Singing wasn't enough of an antidote to the dissatisfaction with work and over the weeks following the Lockerbie plane crash, things eventually came to a head. I was promised that, after two years working as a junior partner on a tenth share of the profits, I would be made a full partner. The three of us would work equally together until both older men retired in the following two years. I was now well into my fourth year, with no sign of full partnership or retirement. They'd been reminded of the handshake that secured our agreement on several occasions, to no effect. Maggie and I needed to move. Neither of us liked living in the city and we didn't want to bring up children here. A single-handed post on Islay – an island in the Inner Hebrides – had come up in the *British Medical Journal.* I knew about it already as it was in the area covered by the Health Board I worked in.

Application forms were sent in and there was a little wait until we discovered we'd been shortlisted from twenty-three other applicants for interview. The next few weeks were a flurry of activity as we planned and eventually made a visit to the practice in Port Ellen, at the southern end of Islay. We sailed out in a gale-blown two-hour crossing, with the two older boys running from one side of the boat to the other as it pitched and rolled. They loved it each time a wave broke over the bow and drenched the lounge in spray, much to the consternation of the other passengers, who were slowly lowering their heads and going green. The whole trip was a success, with both of us feeling a sense of freedom as we looked round the island and the practice. There were nearly 1,200 patients on the list, which was perfect for keeping my skills up, and Maggie would be able to share work with other practices if she wanted. Coming back to work in Glasgow didn't feel like such a burden and the secret I had made me feel more powerful. We were not staying here.

The day after the interview for the post, the phone rang. Sitting in anticipation on the telephone seat, holding the cream handset to my ear, I listened to what was said. I was eager to hear that our freedom was beginning but the tone of his voice was wrong, not upbeat and cheerful, instead quiet, almost sombre. I returned the receiver to its place. In the kitchen, for the first time since I was a child, tears flowed freely as Maggie held on to me. I desperately wanted to get out of here. My whole dream of general practice had been shattered by repetitive care and indifferent colleagues.

The decision had been made – we had to move. We were very definitely in the wrong place for us. Each week I scoured the *British Medical Journal* for other posts, rural posts away from the city routine, and in a place where I could be my own boss. At first, there was a never-ending stream of inner-city practices looking for junior partners.

No on-call but presumably the same stream of work as in my practice. Then, five weeks later, there was an advert from Orkney Health Board for another island practice on an island called Eday. How did you even pronounce that? It said the list size was 125 patients but that must have been a misprint. Surely, it would have to be 1,250 to make it worthwhile having a doctor, to make it worthwhile moving there.

11

Things Unsaid

There were only 125 patients on the practice list and probably a similar number of mice when we first arrived in our new home. Mealtimes are silent now, though, no longer accompanied by the staccato rhythm of mousetraps going off, much to the disappointment of the boys, who were enjoying the chorus of the mousetrap song – 'That's another one gone, Nana, only twenty more to go!' In the few weeks Maggie has been away I've been busy around the house trying to improve it for her return. The holes in the skirtings are full of wire wool and Polyfilla so we haven't seen many mice for a while. New white Artex covers the cracks and crumbles in the walls and Peedie-boot-friendly brown carpet tiles have been laid in the kitchen area. The house is slowly turning around; settling to its new finishes, preparing for a new arrival.

In late May the evening light is strong now, hardly fading until eleven o'clock. The extra light is energizing, mood-lifting, giving the island a whole new life, summer life. There's nearly perpetual daylight, the island resting in the 'simmer dim' only briefly from midnight to two in the morning. I love this light, it gives me energy, reducing my need for sleep. So here I am, twenty feet in the air, holding a five-inch wall brush in one hand, a plastic bucket of whitewash in the other, ready to sort out this grey building while listening to a reading of *Janet and John Went to the Park* rising up from the bottom of the ladder.

Matthew is sitting on the grass, wearing his favourite Lenny the Lion jumper, working his way through his page of reading homework. He is word-perfect, thank goodness, and really quite fast tonight. Is he too fast? The tiny inflections in his voice, the lack of hesitation, the steady rhythm, confident in his words, knowing that they're true. Something doesn't feel right. In medicine there's a lot of talk about intuition. It doesn't exist. Details exists, tiny insignificant fleeting details; like Sherlock Holmes, you have to see, hear, feel all the small things. The finger tightenings, eyelid flickerings, word choosing, rhythms of speech. These things point to the anxieties, tensions, sad half-truths that block diagnosis and mask the deeper stories. Is there something not right? Maybe it's this light making me excited, fanciful, over-imaginative.

Below me in the garden, with all the homework finished now, the boys are running around screaming. The little ones are not quite big enough for a proper game of football, so Martin is being 'big brother' and letting them have shots at him in goal. A snow-white Peedie head chasing a much larger ginger Mikey head, while a tousled fair-headed Matthew waits on a shot at goal. They're doing okay without their mum. They're really a good little team, looking out for each other. I'm proud of them.

Quick strokes with the paintbrush on the rough wall are accompanied by a song in my head. A word I've heard or been thinking about – this time it's 'rhythm' – has done it again and triggered a tune, which is stuck on replay. Sammy Davis Jr's voice, singing 'Rhythm of Life', flows round and round, putting my brain on hold, while each brushstroke picks up the song's beat, as paint flies at the wall.

Rhythm...

'Matthew, come here a minute, pal. Can you read me your story again? I couldn't quite hear all of it up the ladder.'

'Hang on, Dad, 'til I score a goal!'

'Okay, I'll have a seat on the grass.' He's not long scoring and darts across to me.

'Just read the last paragraph for me, I didn't catch it all.'

And he does, word-perfect, quickly, without a single hesitation.

'That's brilliant, can you read the next page, so I can hear more story?'

'But the teacher hasn't read that bit yet!'

'I know, give it a go.'

There it is. He can't read the next sentence. He stumbles and stops and checks and tries and finally stops. The rhythm broken.

'How can you read the first page, pal?'

'The teacher reads it.'

'And?'

'I remember it.'

'How many times does she read it?'

'Once.'

'You remember the whole page after she reads it once to the class, pages without pictures or anything?'

'It's easy, Dad. Can I go and play more football now?'

How people say things is important – gestures with the story, pauses in the rhythm, these are where to look. Chosen words give half the story, between the words lies the truth.

The following day's surgery is busy, everything from signing a request for a shotgun licence to routine prescriptions. Even the minimal prescription charge can be difficult for some people to pay, so I've developed a system of barter. It seems to work well. Noting the name of each patient on the form to go back to the Health

Board, I either place their money in the collection tin or pay it in myself. In return, plastic bags appear, hanging on the new kitchen door, three cabbages at the lower end of the scale, fresh lobster at the upper end. The system is working so well that the boys now regularly ask for lobster for tea! The word 'decadence' comes to mind.

Indeed, decadence has come to the island in the shape of a visitor. Like a swallow, she has migrated north with the spring sunshine, to nest for the summer in the Laird's house. Her accent suggests she comes from the deep south, which proves to be the case when we start the consultation.

Flowing into the room, her tweed Inverness cape swinging behind her, she turns and perches on the edge of the old armchair while, without pausing for breath, telling me she is here to investigate some old manuscripts kept in the Laird's house on Calf Sound. Documents that are too delicate to transport. In a continuous movement, still talking, she delves into an incongruous Louis Vuitton handbag, held firmly in her lap. Finally, she hesitates and presents me, reluctantly, uncertainly, with a letter, unsure if I should be allowed to handle this precious thing. Thick bond paper, watermarked and embossed, lies between my fingertips, the letterhead announcing the name of a skin specialist in Harley Street while the script, in the curt, patronizing language of a specialist writing to a mere general practitioner, details her diagnosis and treatment. Treatment which she has inevitably left in Chelsea. This pretentious, overly ornate letter, with its air of condescension, offends me. It doesn't fit on my island.

'I really must have this medication, Doctor,' she says. 'I know it's unusual but I really would be grateful if you could order it for me.'

Why can some people make a request sound like an order? Carefully reading the letter, my serious consultation face is in place while I inwardly try not to laugh. That would be unfair.

'Let me see what I have in stock,' I say, nipping quickly into my dispensary, coughing.

'No, I don't seem to have any of those pills right enough.'

Reducing the whole letter to 'pills', I bring it into context for the island. On the shelf in front of me are 1,000 yellow tablets exactly matching the prescribed medication from Harley Street.

'Leave it with me and I'll contact my pharmacist and get them flown out specially for you.'

The handbag clicks shut and with a clack of heels on the vinyl floor, off she goes.

Belief in treatment is as important as the treatment itself, so I've not handed her the 'pills' from my island stock. From my patient's viewpoint, she has paid for expensive specialist advice in Harley Street, which she believes in. The letter is carefully preserved, uncreased through her long journey north, giving her confidence while maintaining the connection with Harley Street and her specialist. Perhaps in the past I would have highlighted how smart I was by explaining the simplicity of her condition and the potential cheapness of her treatment, asserting that she doesn't need Harley Street to treat her and countering the offence I felt reading the letter! But that doesn't feel like the right thing to do any more. Having lived on Eday now for nine months, the need to assert myself has become less and less relevant. It's more important for my patient to believe in her physician and his view of the world. I don't need to destroy that relationship in order to fulfil any need of my own ego. The treatment he has prescribed is exactly right, so I maintain her understanding that the medication is unusual, special, through a little subterfuge. Tomorrow, I will take her a month's supply of oxytetracycline (a cheap and common antibiotic) to treat her acne rosacea (a common mild skin condition) and maintain her faith in the expensive and exclusive things of life. There's no need to cause her concern, I can tell she won't be here long enough to learn that exclusivity isn't important.

That evening, high on my painting perch again, hovering above the walled garden, I try to relax a little, letting my gaze drift westward over the thick patch of wild dog rose, to the heather stretching across the peat bog and on to the hillside beyond. The browns and greens are lit by the northern sun, still strong, with no suggestion of sunset this early. It really is beautiful at this time of year with no suggestion of Eday's wild, unpredictable nature. I can feel some of my twisted lines loosen, perhaps straighten a little, as the evening settles on the island.

Slowly, rhythmically, my brush works across the front of the house. Not able to care for Maggie directly, I'm concentrating on caring for the people and things nearest her. Substituting, making things perfect for her return, at the same time aware of being lucky to have all this work to do. She has the hardest work. My mind is filled with 'things' and 'tasks' while she has to settle for crocheting for a baby that still may not come. *If it comes.* Even with all the tasks to occupy me, this thought, preparing for the worst, still lurks insidiously behind everything. At least the house won't be so bad, even if ...

Maggie and I would usually deal with the 'ifs' of life by talking them through together. When my lines get bent, questions are posed: 'Can you do anything about it?' and 'What will change if you worry?' To cope with the distance between us, breaking the hold of the island, I have tried to write to Maggie every second or third evening. Once everyone has gone to bed and the sun lies behind the northern horizon, I write my letter to Maggie. An attempt to share the day's activities and stories so we stay in contact. Even though we chat on the phone in the evening, the letters we send seem more tangible somehow, a fingertip touching over the miles, both holding the same sheets of paper and reinforcing the bond between us.

Crafted late at night with a fountain pen, the letters capture a slice of each day, careful italic script in light blue ink flowing over the page, unhurried even with the lateness of the hour. Each one a collage of events stitched together with clumsy attempts at expressions of love. The envelopes are addressed to Mrs Alexander, not Dr Simpson, Maggie's maiden name. As she said that day we wrote out her maternity card, she has for the moment relinquished the title of 'Doctor' for motherhood. A separate, larger envelope with the drawings and letters from the boys, Mikey's homework taking pride of place, are sent at the same time. I'm not sure why the two envelopes are kept separate, perhaps to preserve a feeling of privacy between us, holding on to the touching. Gripping something fragile.

Despite the letters being held separate from the other things sent south, the stories themselves aren't private. They are simply an attempt to share with Maggie the day-to-day adventures around the house, an attempt at normality, breaking the hold the distance has on us, but there is always an undercurrent, a tidal undertow of anxiety showing in us all. The 'ifs' breaking through, looking for reassurance.

Heatherlea
Eday

Hiya. It's me,

Ah well! Hoped it might be someone handsome, eh! I'm hiding in the front room at the moment. The human tornado is busy in the kitchen. Did you know a mouse had been in the pot cupboard?? It's been well and truly gutted – the cupboard, not the mouse, although that may follow if I can't rescue it. I think the mice know Nana is here. We sat at supper in the kitchen while they danced under the bathroom floor! Nana is well, as you can tell.

Mary phoned tonight and was pleased to hear you were feeling better. I don't always give the full picture on the phone.

Peedie seems back to normal. He ate four helpings of the rice pudding I made. Even Nana seemed to approve of it and ate a fair helping. Even if it did have two small black bits in it. Probably mouse droppings from the pot cupboard!!

Pots, mice, phone calls and rice pudding, an eclectic mix for one day. Nana, Maggie's mum, is held on the island just as much as I am. She copes with the stress by cleaning – anything and everything, even if it has been cleaned before. A human tornado whipping up everything in front of her, paying attention to the physical, never the emotional. She never speaks about anything worrying her, she simply increases her work rate to deal with increasing anxiety. There's a little frisson of disapproval in this extract, where I let my annoyance at Nana's inability to express herself come through. Almost hoping that the 'two small black bits' are indeed mouse droppings and not burned rice.

Heatherlea
Eday

Hello, I'm back,

Not much of a day, is it? We've tried to wrap up your coffee buns in an indestructible fashion but you'll probably just receive a box of crumbs. You can sweep them up and eat them.

I've got Mother sneezing even more with my sanding of the banister. I was hoping to cut peat this afternoon but couldn't because of the rain. Anyway, the stair is coming on slowly, I'm nearly ready to start painting. I'll try to lighten the pink and see how it looks.

The goat's milk is much better now and almost as good as before. The boys are drinking it readily. I've to make cheese tomorrow. The last lot was quite good but it was hung for three days. Plenty of duck eggs still, so may make ice cream soon. Got into trouble for eating your coffee buns today but pinched another when she wasn't looking.

Everyone continues to ask for you, Carol was in today but I didn't get a chance to ask about the beds.

Peedie is settling down and stays happily with Nana now. He's even started to diagnose now. When someone went into the surgery, Nana said they had a sore tummy, Peedie said, 'No, sore head!' He was probably more accurate than I was. Did a two-and-a-half-hour surgery this morning. Nana thought I'd died in there.

Well, not much more happened today so I'll go and pop this into your food parcel.

Keep going, we'll make it. Just think, with all this cooking practice you won't have to cook 'til Christmas.

Love you (that word doesn't seem big enough, try again!)

LOVE YOU (that's better)

'Keep going, we'll make it.' *If it comes.* That thought creeping into the last line then discarded with a joke about cooking. Reaching out to give and get reassurance over the miles. A brief recognition, a touching of the anxiety, the unspoken question in the middle of everything. Life is a strange mixture of hunger and burst. Too many eggs, too much milk, suddenly busy surgeries. Then spells where I consider going to cut peat or make cheese. Being the doctor on the island isn't anything like the city practice we're both used to. On the island you are available all the time, night and day, ready to drop everything and go, but more importantly, it is about fitting into the pattern of the island. Settling on to the surface and being part of the structure. This means learning to make cheese, cutting peat, gathering eggs and making ice cream. Folk watch these things and agree among themselves that you are suitable, that you will do as a family and as a doctor. Each element as important as the other.

Heatherlea

Eday

It's that man again,

Started to shift peat today in an attempt to improve the TV signal. If I move enough peat I should make a hole in the hill and let the signal through. I've had advice from Erland and Arthur, so I can't go wrong. Matthew was a tremendous help and stacked peats like a Trojan. Martin, I think, stacked five peats all day. Michael 'tinkled' on as many peats as he could. Peedie now shouts 'Geronimo' and throws himself into the peat bog. I left him home in the afternoon. I'll have to put sun cream on Michael tomorrow.

I've given Nana her homeopathic Rhus Tox today, so I hope it works. She did take it quite religiously at the right times.

Michael is drinking gallons of milk and Matthew has decided he likes Ribena in it. Martin screws his face up. I think Martin is needing more homeopathic therapy too and I wonder if sulphur may be more appropriate. I'll think about it.

That's good news about your method of delivery. Sounds as though the specialist will do all right by you. I can probably be with you readily on Monday the 4th of June. Nana says she could watch the boys in Kirkwall. We'll keep it in mind. I'd like to be there if at all possible. Obviously the peedies' welfare will have to come first.

Erland was in tonight to see if a change in his Sinemet could improve his Parkinson's symptoms and make him better at cutting peats. I said if he cut them any better the hill would collapse, which he seemed to appreciate.

Well, I'll stop now. Less news today because we have been out all day. I'll write tomorrow but we hit the weekend hiccup in the post.

Still love you very much (thought it might wear off by now, eh!).

P.S. Still haven't got your letter yet – hope it comes tomorrow.

Little stresses and fractures detailed in a few words. Martin becoming more upset, not helping with the peat cutting, screwing his face up, all out of character. Nana needing her homeopathic therapy to help with her arthritis, aggravated by overwork. I pretend these letters are light and newsy but the need to touch base with Maggie, to detail the truth, is still there.

Against this backdrop of disruption, of dislocation, we're settling into the rhythm of the island, being accepted at the peat cutting, even if it is done badly at first.

The peat bank for the doctor's house is immediately behind the house at the foot of the hill. There are three banks in that bit of bog, one for Erland, one for Arthur and the other for the doctor. I had spent the winter trying to find out which bank is mine but no one would tell me and I couldn't understand why not. All I got was vague responses along the lines of 'Aye, over there, Doc' or 'Just right behind the house'. I have decided to take matters into my own hands and have gone out with my spade to start hacking at a likely bank. I reckoned if it was the wrong bank, folks would be quick to tell me. I picked the correct bank and after that Erland and Arthur, both in their seventies, have been quick to help me and show me how to cut properly – Erland perhaps hoping that my lesson in the winter on how peat should be stacked has been learned. It has also become apparent that if I hadn't cut the bank this year then I would have lost the right to do so. Any bank left uncut for three consecutive years is up for grabs. These particular banks are 'black peat' banks, in short supply on the island, the very best form of burning peat, rich in oils and extremely hard once they are dried. It's important I cut them well, not just for Erland and Arthur, but for the watching eyes driving past on the island road.

It's nearly 1 a.m. now and I'm sitting down to write to Maggie again. It's still light enough to see to write if I sit near the window. Somehow putting the electric light on seems like an intrusion on the peace of the night. The shore music plays all night now, curlews and oystercatchers mingling with the sounds of the waves, while the peewits' sing-song call sounds across the fields, joining the chorus from the shore. I managed to stop Nana from cleaning today and took her out on visits with me. We saw swallows feeding over the tangles – the seaweed – on Warness Beach while the sea lay peacefully along the shore, glass-like, the blue surface breathing gently in the afternoon sun. She approved of the tidy stacks of seaweed stalks that had been ripped from the seabed in the winter storms, now piled on to racks at the top of the beach, drying in the summer winds. Each ton of stalks is ready to be sent off to pharmaceutical companies to be processed. It was good to see them cleaned off the beach, she said.

On afternoons like that you imagine you can easily row a boat to Kirkwall, the only disturbances in the water are eddies pushed up by hidden rocks, as the tide ebbs and flows across them. These hidden forces cannot be changed, only accepted. Allowing yourself to go with the rhythm, with the flow they create. Far out beyond the headland there was a figure standing up in a tiny rowing boat. A man standing on the water surface, hauling in creels, with currents flowing around him, tiny, insignificant in the huge sea around him. In control and vulnerable simultaneously.

Maggie and I have seen the other side of this sea, when deep-sea trawlers disappear for minutes on end in the troughs of the waves as they course through the sound. I'm very aware of not taking anything for granted. Just as the sea's mood can change unpredictably, driven by wind and tide, life can turn too. *If it comes.* There's good news now, though. Maggie's specialist thinks the placenta is moving up a little, away from the neck of the womb. He will allow Maggie a 'trial of labour'. There's still a risk of bleeding during labour and an emergency section is still possible but this will be in a safer hospital environment. Perhaps I should let myself relax and allow the 'ifs' to drift away a little.

Living and Dying

I am Eid-ey,
The isthmus isle, the connector of tidal lands.

Before man I was and after man I will be.
Men with stones, men with iron, farmers
and sea gatherers
have bruised my land for millennia.
Still they come
with new ideas as Old as my stones.
They think they change
but they do not.
Living and Dying remain the same.

12

Deep Roots

The dentist has arrived for his annual visit. I hadn't really thought about dentistry and how that could happen on the island. He has asked to use my surgery as it's the only clinical space. I've cancelled this morning's surgery to let him have the space and already a small queue is forming in the waiting room. Before he starts, Mr Cameron sits with us in the kitchen, quietly supping a cup of tea. In contrast to Trevor, my locum, who is always quite dapper in appearance, Mr Cameron looks as though dressing was an afterthought. His clothes are lumpy, thick wool and tweed fitting only where it touches. There's a shyness about him and, like many Orcadian men, a reluctance to conversation that belies the fact that they have any opinions. Opinions must be carefully shared and not on first meetings. Initial meetings are polite, with a reserve that can be taken for rudeness until you understand the ways of working. Even a handshake will at times be taken as too forward, a simple nod of the head will suffice and a murmured 'Aye'. He deliberately hands me a large box of chocolates 'for my wife', as he says. A thank you for our hospitality and the free use of the surgery. I doubt if the chocolates will survive until Maggie comes home from Aberdeen. Nana has a sweet tooth.

'Will I call you if I see anything interesting today?' he asks quietly before going through to his work.

'Aye, that would good. I don't know anything about dentistry,' I say in return.

'I could show you how to pull a tooth if you like, there's sure to be some needing done.'

'Give me a shout if you do. I'll not be far away today.'

True to his word, he calls me through in the early afternoon. Willick needs a tooth pulled.

'I can't fill teeth out here,' Mr Cameron tells me. 'Mr Flaws would need to come into Kirkwall to let me do that.'

'Isn't there a dental van that comes around?'

'There used to be in the 1960s but it got too heavy to winch on to the *Orcadia* latterly. So now I go around the isles and do what I can.'

With that, he continues to prepare Willick for the extraction. I am not a great fan of obstetric instruments – the Wrigley's forceps are still firmly shut in the drawer – but it looks like I may have to add dental implements to my avoidance list as well. My desk is covered in steel pliers, probes and syringes. I have a fanciful idea that he may be about to heat a needle in methylated spirit flame to sterilize it until I remember that image is from my childhood TB vaccine.

'Can you hold his head, please, just to make him comfortable.'

'You okay, Willick?' I ask.

Willick nods slightly and shrugs his shoulders, as Mr Cameron brings the pliers up to his mouth. I've never been squeamish at surgical operations, I just find the process of surgery boring, the puzzle being already solved, leaving only the mechanics of removal and repair. Performing medical techniques like bone marrow aspiration, thoracic drain insertion, lumber puncture is much more interesting, as you're looking for clues, markers as to the causes of illness. Those tasks require three-dimensional awareness and a little bravery as you insert a needle or tube into someone, all the time trying in your mind's eye to see the way forward, imagine where you are. Perhaps one day someone will invent a safe scan that allows me to see 'real time' where the needle point is but for now I make do with a detailed knowledge of anatomy and courage. Courage, however, seems to fail me as I watch the pliers grab the offending tooth with a very slight but perceptible crunch, while the unholy effort of freeing the offending item begins. Orcadian men seem to have deep roots. I have to look away until the struggle is over, simultaneously making a mental note to never again refer to anything difficult as 'like pulling teeth'.

'It's probably more useful if you know how to stop dental haemorrhage than pull teeth,' says Mr Cameron as he rattles the offending tooth into a silver kidney dish on my desk. Meanwhile, Willick spits blood into the old nylon basin we use for cleaning the surgery. 'Basically, you just need pressure on the socket most times. Get them to bite down on to a rolled-up swab and hold it there for half an hour if they can. That should do it. Sometimes we soak the swab in adrenalin, but you need to watch what you're doing with that. Have you an ECG machine?'

'No, not yet anyway. Hopefully we'll have one next week.'

'That's good. You're first in the Isles to have one, I think.'

'I think so. I decided we needed one after I had a patient with angina I wanted to monitor and couldn't.'

'Right, Mr Flaws,' he says, looking down at Willick and his basin of blood. 'You're good to go. No dram for you tonight or tomorrow and leave the Laird's garden alone for a day or two as well. We don't want you bleeding, do we?'

Once Willick has left the surgery, Mr Cameron turns to me again.

'These old boys are tough as nails, but they also think they're indestructible. It's difficult to get them to take things easy after extraction. If you get a chance, could you look in on him tomorrow and see if he's behaving himself?'

The next morning I stop at Willick's house near the shore on Calf Sound, the gatehouse to the Laird's eighteenth-century family dwelling. The grass around his grey cottage is neatly trimmed, as are the paths leading to the stony seashore and the Loch of Carrick a hundred yards away. As I walk up to the cottage a loon, a red-throated diver, flies overhead, going out to sea to fish. Its creaking, rasping 'leaving' call follows it as it goes. The windows to Willick's cottage are undressed and blank, giving the place a sullen, uninviting look. Looking closely through the glass I can see a sparsely furnished sitting room, devoid of decoration apart from an ash-coated peat stove. The peat dust spills on to the bare floor. A circle of brown 'yarfe' peat lies around a galvanized bucket, an evening's supply of the poorer burning brown peat cut from higher up the island hillsides. Bare walls match the floors, continuing the sense of emptiness in the building. I'm used to homes being relatively uniform down south, large estates of similar houses giving little away about the individual inhabitants. Here the houses are an extension of the people, unfettered by any social pressures, reflecting the folks living there. Willick's precisely cut grass pathways lead to practical places like the shore and the loch side. Unnecessary decoration or adornment is clearly pointless in his eyes. Functionality is key. Just as I turn away from the window, there's a slight movement behind me.

'Aye, Doctor.' The two words are given the power of censure at my intrusion.

'Ah, Willick, how are you today?'

'Fine.'

'It's just ... well ... Mr Cameron asked me to look in and check on your tooth.'

'Why?'

'To make sure it wasn't bleeding and to see if you ...'

Courage fails me for the second time in two days as I decide not to ask whether he's resting. He's dressed in his familiar blue padded boiler suit, the only clothes I've ever seen him wear. Two plastic Co-operative Food Store bags hang at his side, weighted with vegetables from the Laird's garden. The legs of the boiler suit and the black Wellington boots sticking out the bottom are completely covered in grass clippings.

'Shall we go inside?' I say, hoping to recover some control of the conversation as I turn towards the door.

When I reach for the door handle, I realize that Willick hasn't followed me. Looking back, he's still standing defiantly immobile on the path with his mouth wide open. Admitting defeat, I rummage in my bag for a torch, which I shine pointlessly into his mouth. Even if the tooth socket is oozing blood I doubt if I can persuade him to rest.

My next visit is to Frank Cottlestone, just along the shore from Carrick House. As I stop the car on the gravel driveway outside the neat, flagstone-roofed little house, I decide I've had enough of them this time. Each visit I've made here has resulted in the two Jack Russell terriers sneaking up on me and grabbing my trouser legs or worse. Looking out from the car, they are nowhere in sight. They are always nowhere in sight! Waiting to make their clandestine attacks from within the thick *Rosa rugosa* bushes or from behind the low walls surrounding the property. The colourful plantings of alpines and heathers along the top of the low walls always distracts me, making me forget about the canine menace.

Taking my medical case from the boot of the car, I set off along the path to the house. Just as I'm about to round the corner of the building there's a telltale scuffling of feet and just a hint of the attack yap. Executing my pre-planned manoeuvre, I swing my case briskly behind me and feel it connect satisfyingly with a presumably already open set of jaws. This is followed by a duet of yelping – my aim was better than I had hoped for. Casually turning to see what the noise was, I spot two fast-moving canine rear ends disappearing into the thick wild roses.

'Morning, Doc,' says Mr C. 'Did you see the dogs this morning? They've not been around for a while.'

'I think I just missed them,' I lie. 'I saw them disappearing into the rose bushes a moment ago.'

Mr C's garden is immaculate, as he's sculpted and shaped the walls of the ruined buildings around the cottage into individual garden areas. These fall in steps and stairs down to the shore of Calf Sound, protecting the low-lying plants from the worst of the winter weather. Here, even ground-level plants can get battered in a good gale. His artist's eye has created an idyllic scene looking north to the steep cliffs of the Red Head on one side and the island to the north – the Calf of Eday – on the other. As we sit outside and talk, the fast tidal race flows through the narrows of Calf Sound, setting up standing waves in the centre of the stream. A fishing boat rests along the north shore of the sound. Cleverly anchored 6 feet outside the tidal race, it swings quietly on its anchor chain, unperturbed by the torrent beside it. So much of living well in this place is about learning to work with the elements. Pushing against them doesn't work but that doesn't mean you can't shape and meld them to your purposes.

13

Swan Song

Having survived an intoxicating episode driven by greed in January this year, our gander Albert has been in trouble again. He managed to escape from the paddock on to the road and has sustained a nasty injury to his head and a broken beak after running in front of a car. We tried to keep him in the hospital shed at first, but he is far too feisty for that nonsense and, like the good Orcadian male he now is, he's up and in the field again. This incident, coupled with the increasing need to keep our new goats in the paddock, has meant that I need a new fence. Not that a new fence will necessarily stop the goats escaping, as anyone who has lived with them will know. Goats seem to have a similar ability to mice and are able to completely flatten their chests on to the ground and commando crawl under ludicrously low fences. This, in combination with their 'springability', makes them almost impossible to keep in. Anyway, I should try to contain them, not least because we're right beside the main road, which can be extremely busy on delivery Wednesday, when the supply boat comes in. Sometimes there are two cars every ten minutes.

As June begins to consider the possibility of summer, the days lengthen even further and there's time to look for help with erecting the fence. Most folks have finished cutting and stacking the peats and rows of tiny henges, three peats for the base with a fourth laid across as a roof, wait on hillsides for the summer winds to shrink and harden them as they dry. It's a technique perfected by years of experience. The grass is only just thinking about lifting its head into the gentler summer wind and hasn't grown sufficiently yet to cut for hay or silage. There's a very brief slack period when I could get help with setting a new fence in place. Having mentioned my plan to Rob, he volunteered to come and drill the strainer post holes for me with his tractor. He has an augur attachment which can be driven from the prop shaft and is able to make short work of preparing the holes. It's essentially a corkscrew for making holes in fields.

A week later and just as I'm finishing Saturday morning's breakfast dishes, I realize that Rob has started work. The manner he has adopted isn't quite what I had expected as I watch out the kitchen window. I'm fairly sure that the rear wheels of the tractor aren't supposed to be coming off the ground. All I can see at the moment is the old Massey Ferguson rising slowly into the air at the bottom end of the paddock. Rob's face is just visible, with its huge bushy black beard, and he seems to be levitating too! Now, I'm not an expert in matters tractor but I'm pretty sure that re-enacting the ascension of Elijah wasn't really part of the plan.

He may have been overconfident in thinking the ground would be soft, fooled by how close the house is to the peat banks. It's bound to be an easy job. An hour has passed, and the tractor now appears to have taken on the role of a bucking bronco from some bizarre rodeo. Rob is now just a blur of beard and bobble hat waving about in the sky. I think his pipe, usually clamped firmly between his teeth, may have vanished into the heather. I'm not aware of rodeo being part of the Orkney County Show activities but if it is then Rob – even as an incomer – clearly has a chance of gold.

Now, Orcadians can be many things but one thing they are not is stupid. There is no way they would have allowed the Health Board to actually build the doctor's house in a peat bog. Not least because it would make it terribly inconvenient for driving to the surgery. The house is built where a house should be built, on rock. It is also built at the top of a hill, which, incidentally, Orcadians wouldn't do either, because of the wind. That, however, is a mere detail as I've now learned wind never stopped an

Orcadian from doing anything. Rob, too, has discovered that Orcadians are clever people and he has just rung the doorbell. He looks considerably shaken but has at least recovered his pipe, which is firmly fixed into its familiar spot in his beard.

The pipe is one of the curved stem types with a large gnarled bowl, and it sits in the only brown bit of his shaggy beard, an area that has obviously taken time and effort to mature. The pipe wags up and down, mesmerizing me, as he explains the problems he's encountered. He's a kind man and is visibly upset that he can't help me. Part of the essence of island life is bartering in kindnesses: one day I'll do something to help you and no doubt, at some point in the future, you'll do me a return favour. There's no contract or bill of sale, just an understanding that when all is said and done, we need each other if we are to survive fifteen miles out to sea.

It doesn't take long for word to get around that the doctor may have some work needing done. Monday morning, just after surgery finishes around 11 a.m., Willick knocks on the kitchen door. Did the doctor need a peedie bit of fencing done? He'd heard at the Co-op that I'd ordered a load of fence posts and wire from Scarth's on the mainland.

One of many things I've had to get used to living on such a small island is the concept of privacy. Privacy applies to personal things like feelings and emotions.

Practical things like who's having a baby, who's thinking about moving house, or who might need a little bit of paid work done, these things are not private. These things have practical implications and so are communal. A new baby will mean a child at school in due course, keeping the island school alive. Moving house will mean a day's work for some of the men and so on. So Willick has heard there may be work at the doctor's and here he is. Not to offer himself for the work, though, as he's in his seventies now. No, his younger cousin Ivan is a fine fencer and he would gladly do it. Ivan is only in his sixties, so is clearly fit to do the job. I point out the difficulties Rob had with the ground but that doesn't faze Willick. His cousin will dig the holes for the strainers by hand.

Early on Tuesday morning, before I've had a chance to think about house calls, Ivan is here to start work. I never heard him arrive. Usually, you hear the cars draw up long before someone rings the bell but he has little time for cars and has walked to Heatherlea over the hill, carrying his tools. As we stand and talk in the yard I realize something else. I've never seen him before! He's never been to the surgery and I've never seen him at the two other meeting places, the shop and the pier. As we talk through the job to be done it soon becomes clear why we haven't met before. Ivan is painfully shy and quiet. His head falls forward as he speaks in soft accented tones but his eyes stay with you. Watching you, gauging the effect of his words, measuring the distance between you and him. If he's comfortable he'll work with you, if not he won't. When I ask why I've not seen him before at the shop or elsewhere, he slowly shrugs his shoulders and says he only visits the shop on a quiet day, making sure to order all the goods likely to be in short supply ahead of time.

We walk around the paddock and agree the layout of the fence and the necessary positions of the thick strainer posts. Strainer posts are the big round posts that you see at corners of fields looking like short telegraph poles. They are eight feet long and need to be sunk into the ground for a good three feet if they are to do their job properly. They literally take the strain of the fence wire.

I had expected Ivan to have an array of pickaxes, pinch bars and other rock-digging implements. Perhaps even some Second World War dynamite, given Rob's tractor experience. But no. He has a decent long-handled cutting spade, which is heart-shaped and sharp, and a double spade. A double spade is exactly as the name suggests. It is two long-handled spades joined by a scissor-type connection that allows you to lift earth and stone from the bottom of the hole. Having tried to dig the ground myself, I'm sceptical how these will work.

The morning is surprisingly busy so I forget about Ivan until lunchtime. Nana has made some soup, so I wander across to invite him to come in and warm up, and have some lunch. He refuses to come in. Even when I point out that there's rain coming he remains determined to stay outside. He'll be perfectly all right in the goat shed until it passes, as it surely will. There's no way I can persuade him, so I turn to leave. It's only then I notice the deep hole in the ground beyond the shed. Nearly three feet deep by just a foot and half wide. Ideal for a strainer post. How did he do that? No point in asking, he'll just give me a shy smile.

The next day is quieter and I'm determined to try to see how these holes are dug. Four holes are complete now. Sitting on the old sagging fence, I watch the swift, accurate descent of the long-handled spade, cutting the outline of a new hole, followed by the removal of the fibrous turf. There's no apparent muscular effort in the careful, deliberate strokes, only a synergy between man and spade persuading the earth to give way. The secret seems to be in the flow of the action, not brute force. Slowly the spade goes deeper, further into the earth, followed by pauses while Ivan bends down to ease stones from the soil with his hands. Why haven't I noticed his hands before now? Coarse brown skin covers them, not ingrained with dirt but simply showing years of labour in all weathers. Strong fingers impervious to the sharp rocks, obviating the need for leather gloves. Then, once the hole is deep enough, the change to the double spade. One hand on each spade handle as it's driven down into the earth, the handles pulled apart then closed as rock and earth are lifted out. Slowly and methodically, the earth gives way, allowing the positioning of the posts. I've seen other farmers elsewhere using JCBs to dig post holes and adding special attachments to pile-drive in the posts. Here in my paddock is how it's been done for years without the use of hydraulic machines. In fact, the post holes are being dug when machines couldn't! I suppose I'm watching an expression of the resilience of islanders everywhere. Getting things done with the minimum fuss.

I never manage to get Ivan to chat, though. In the whole week it has taken him to set the fence he's only ever exchanged polite good mornings and refusals to come in for a cup of tea. Words, language aren't a necessary thing for him. He seems to regard them as an intrusion on the world around, noise that displaces the peace of the place we're in. Sitting on the grass with our backs to the stone wall of the garden, we shelter from the wind and survey the new fence as I hand him his payment for the job. Below us, Mill Loch lies quiet and undisturbed, with the exception of the cries of the loons as they meet up with their mates again, ready to establish their nests for this year. There are times when words are superfluous; sometimes company is enough.

I'm still finding living near the top of the world has plenty to teach me. Maggie is very keen on being eco-friendly, so we have always had terry towelling nappies for our babies. Peedie is almost out of nappies but he still needs one at night time. These need to be steeped, washed and dried but that's not difficult up here on the hill where the summer wind is plentiful and at times overabundant. There's nothing better than seeing a full washing line of pristine white nappies blowing in the summer breeze. Lately, however, the wind must be getting stronger or we're needing new nappies as they are beginning to fray at the ends. This can happen of course in the wintertime, when the winds are really strong, but it's not been that windy lately. I've been out to check the washing line and the surroundings and there's nothing to snag the nappies that I can see. Ah well! Better order up some new ones.

On Thursday mornings I've been taking a little time to myself and walking the shores of the island, places I can't readily take the boys. I think I'll continue my walk along the west shore this morning and see if I can find more signs of otter movement. There's a track over Stennie Hill that is definitely a dog otter path, which I'll follow. As I walk along the side of the paddock to head over the hill I notice a single brown trumpet-shaped goat's ear appear round the shed door. Rhoda, our new long-legged Anglo-Nubian goat is checking the air for rain. She is, like all goats, allergic to rain, so careful checking is necessary before venturing out. Next comes her nose, nostrils pulsating as she sniffs the atmosphere for molecules of water. She has a perfect nose for this job as it's slightly bent to the right in a graceful curve. This allows her to sniff round corners. It also allows her to lift latches on gates if needed but that's another story. Today it's a fine day and out she trots with Freda, her bouncy snowball-white kid, springing behind her. Making directly for my new fence, Rhoda, without any apparent effort, leans precisely on the midpoint between two fence posts and stretches the wire as far as it can go. Then, extending her neck, she carefully catches the edge of a pristine white nappy in her teeth and proceeds to chew steadily. No wonder the edges are frayed! Freda, meantime, has run sideways in a graceful arc along the face of the drystane dyke that marks the top of the paddock and clears the new fence without even looking. She is bouncing around below the washing like a pom pom on a pogo stick. As I may have mentioned, attempting to fence in goats is pointless. Poor Ivan, all that effort for nothing.

About five hundred yards along the road from the house, I've picked up the trail going under the fence. The coarse grass plastered against the fence wire by the winter wind has been tunnelled through and the track beneath is worn smooth into an otter-sized run. There are no footprints or drag marks from a tail to make me certain this is what I'm looking for but on the opposite side of the road there are clear signs of the trail extending north towards Mill Loch. I'll follow the southward trail over the hill above the airstrip. It's not easy walking as I am just above the peat bank now, so it's a bit of a scramble over the still brown heather and grassy tussocks, as I guess the route to the shore. I love the feeling as I arrive at the edge of the sea just south of Newark Bay. There's never anybody here and the freedom is immensely relaxing. The water is beautiful today, an acrylic mix of blues and greens, like an artist's palette, the colours all swirling together.

Waiting and watching. Not for anything in particular. I'm just allowing the wind and waves to gently unwind me. It's one of the ways to survive twenty-four hours on call, day after day, for months on end. Beneath me, oystercatchers pepper the shore black and white, while on the hill behind me the plaintive call of peewits echoes my childhood in the Pentland Hills. In one peewit tumbling wing beat, I'm a small boy stretched out once more in the heather, being warmed by the sun, watching the world fall backwards over my head and listening to the birds twist and dive over the fields. The air breathes in time with me as it ebbs and flows through the coarse heather stalks. This is close to where the heart gives out.

Beneath me my childhood village bustle: people walking between Mrs Slimmand's, the fruitmonger, and Archibald's grocery store; the coal lorry making weekly deliveries; the fishmonger's van stopping on the village green, horn sounding to signal his arrival. Occasionally, I would see Dr MacKenzie walking along the street, still clutching his brown Gladstone bag as he went from house to house on his visits. It never occurred to me to think about what he did when he wasn't working. He always seemed to be working. We're more similar now, he and I, than I would have thought possible. When I was a boy, my only aim was to gain entrance to medical school. I don't remember thinking about what it would be like to be a doctor day in, day out.

We don't spend enough time truly doing nothing these days. Especially down south, there always seemed to be another thing to do, a distraction, an invitation to make more of your life. You were validated by the groups and activities you joined. You didn't play your full part if you didn't 'take part'. The island will teach you how to slow down if you let it. Let your heart rest, ease you down from the frenetic and teach you how to simply 'be'. So many incomers still try to make living here what they think it 'should be', spending their time fighting against the rhythm and trying to make the island conform to their way of thinking. They don't last long! They say if you last two winters on the island then you'll stay a while, accepting that you have to bend with the wind.

Further along the shore I can see a suggestion of white on one of the rocks. I'm looking for otter spraint, the little pile of fish bones and guano that they use to mark territory. The bones are mainly from butterfish, a shore-feeding otter's favourite food. Butterfish are remarkably adapted to living on the seashore and even survive stranding when the sea goes out, as they can breathe air through their gills. They hide from predators in thick seaweed or under stones and wait for the tide to come in again. There have been several that didn't avoid predators, however, as this white mark on the rock is definitely a spraint mark. I need to look around carefully now for other signs. I'm looking for a holt mouth or a daytime lie-up called a couch. It will be somewhere against the sandy bank and the rocks. After thirty minutes of searching the shore, I've only been able to find another definite trail leading back towards the airstrip. There is a male otter around here somewhere, patrolling his fiefdom, but I won't see him today.

Wait and watch. Reclaiming the hillside again, I like to sit and watch the Loganair plane come in to land. It is reassuring to see it arrive, my lifeline to the outside world. I'm in luck: as I lie back once more on my springy heather hammock, the plane swings north to land into the southerly breeze. There's just a hiss of air as the plane swoops over my head, propellers idling, spinning backwards slowly in the wind as Dave glides in to land. The landing is tricky from the north, the steep hill falling down to the flat sandy grass below. Nice to watch from up here all the same, a bit like a swan coming down on to a lake. A little ungainly in the crosswinds as air spills from the wings, making it slip from side to side then pull up sharply at the last second before hitting the surface.

As I watch the plane taxi towards the red wooden sheds, there is a sense of something being not right. I'd forgotten what day it is. The plane isn't due until later. The feeling is confirmed when two policemen step out of the plane to be met by the local special constable. These are not traffic police on a fool's errand; this looks more serious as they cluster together with intent looks on their faces. It can't be medical, or they would have paged me to help. I've never actually been completely out of touch, you see, just not immediately able to answer the phone.

Walking back to the house, a bad feeling settles in my stomach. The coastguard pickup truck has just driven north and several other cars appear to be gathering at the shop. Claire's car is abandoned in front of our house too. Not that that is bad in itself; nobody really parks a car here, there's not a need for it. I slip my boots off and push open the door to the kitchen, the smell of cigarette smoke in the porch swirling around and following me inside. Claire doesn't usually smoke when she's at the surgery.

The kitchen is tense and quiet. Nana is standing at the window looking for me, with her cup of tea wrapped protectively in both hands. Claire sits on the edge of the seat, ready to go for another smoke. Ivan is missing, no one has seen him for over a day and, although he's shy, he's not reclusive. He was due to work on one of the westside farms yesterday but didn't turn up. This morning there was no sign of breakfast or even tea dishes left over from last night when they dropped by his house to see him.

Joining the gathering group of island folks at the shop, the sense of apprehension is increasing. Ivan is pretty regular in his habits, so things don't look good. Questions dance from mouth to mouth. Has he fallen and injured himself? Is he stuck on the shore somewhere? Has he left the island? There are parts of this small island which very few folks visit, where you can be alone for days if you choose to be. I've just come back from one. Gradually the questions subside and the search parties form. There's no question of him leaving the island without someone knowing. It's not possible. Even if you had your own boat, someone would see you. He must be on the island somewhere.

The main search is coordinated by the coastguard, just like it would be on any island or coastal community. The difference here is it's the same folks who are the fire brigade and who will become the ambulance crew if I need one. A coastal search is underway and there are people walking the hill paths to see if Ivan is up there. There are good tracks across the island that were used to bring peat down from the hills. Magnus, the special constable, has taken his fishing boat out, sailing from its mooring in Calf Sound around the Red Head to the west side to view the remote shores nearest Ivan's house. I've been sent back to Heatherlea to wait. They need to know where I am quickly, so it's best I stay in one place.

At times like this, the whole community becomes quiet. There's no question of folk not knowing what's happening, the connections are ingrained in the fabric of the island. It's as if we are all one person feeling the same feelings of anxiety and concern. Faced with the possibility of bad news, I go to check what we know about Ivan from his medical records. Nothing. His record is blank. The old brown Lloyd George envelope pocket has only two brown continuation cards in it with nothing written on them. There's not even a record of his vaccinations because he was born before the NHS started and army service vaccinations aren't transferred to NHS cards. I'm not surprised though. He's not the kind of man to come to the doctor. I've nothing useful to add then.

No matter what the search teams find, there are only two of us here to deal with it. I can't call for an ambulance or rapid response unit from the hospital to come and assist. Whatever comes our way we have to deal with, potentially for days if the weather's bad, until we can transport our patient to hospital. I've slowly been building up the equipment since we arrived. We have oxygen for twenty-four hours in bottles, intravenous fluids to cover a similar timeframe, including plasma expanders, which are the nearest we can get to blood should we need it. If someone isn't breathing for themselves, we can manually support them with ambu-bags. Should that need to be for a long time, then we would have to take turns. There's a reasonable range of emergency drugs if we need them, too. Everything seems to be in order. In fact, I knew that before I started to check. I do this every week. I just need to feel I am doing something useful.

It isn't always possible to wait and watch, sometimes I have to fiddle pointlessly.

I spend the night waiting for the phone to ring. Some nights are like that, you get used to the half-sleep nights. Forcing yourself to stick to the routine. Locking up the house, eating supper, stoking the little stove and closing it down for the night. Then making your way to bed, all the time expecting the phone to ring, almost urging it to ring so you can get the problem over with. Eventually, sleep comes but never deeply, just a light doze that lets you answer the phone after the first ring, speaking clearly – 'Dr Alexander' – or so you think until the caller says – 'Sorry, Doctor, did I wake you?' Tonight there is no caller.

The waiting and watching ends. They've found him. When I go through to have morning coffee after surgery, a policeman has just arrived with Magnus. They found him a few minutes ago not far from the surgery, on the hill above Mill Loch. Following Magnus up the road, we stop beside a field track that leads to a gate set back from the road. The damp greyness of the day settles round us as we walk a little way up the path. To the right there's a little cutting dug into the hillside, hidden from view from the road, deep and sheltered from the weather. Looking back down the track, the cutting would be easily missed by searchers on the road. Even the wind can't reach into the hollow and probably Ivan has used this in the past to allow the worst of a squall to pass over before making his way home. He's lying curled up as if he's asleep but he's so cold to touch it's clear he's not. I kneel by him for a minute out of respect, as the wind eases briefly to allow the liquid, lonely call of a loon on the loch below to rise up to us on the hill. Mourning the loss. There is a sadness in the sound, a desolation that is uncomfortable as the long drawn-out notes reflect up to us from the water's surface. I'm not upset that Ivan died on the hill, I don't think that would have bothered him. It is the loneliness of the moment that unsettles me.

There's nothing more for me to do now. The police will have to arrange a post-mortem examination in Kirkwall, so I've just come home. Our two younger boys know that something serious has happened but they're too small to really understand. The older ones will hear at the school before they get back. I don't suppose I think much about the effect these events have on them but it must do, living in the midst of all the moods of the island. They've all known almost from birth what confidentiality is and never ask about events or phone calls. They just accept that there are things that are not spoken about. I don't think that bothers them. What does bother them is when I say we're going to the beach and then the phone rings and all of a sudden we're not any more. The intrusion of being on-call affects meal times and trips surprisingly frequently. It's a way of life really, you could never do it just as a job. It's a way of life for all of us.

A week later, and I'm standing in the middle of the airstrip at the bottom of the hillside where I watched the plane glide in to land. Stan phoned in his role as airport manager this time, to say there's a swan on the airstrip and they can't get it to move. It looks sick. Anything that is sick on the island still seems to default to me. I was asked a while back, by one of the farmers, completely out of the blue, if I was a trained surgeon. I said I had a very basic training, but I wasn't a surgeon. Could I do caesarian sections? No, why? Ah, I couldn't do a caesarian on a cow then? It seems that if a cow gets into difficulties during labour then it's too expensive to call the vet out to do the operation as it can involve hiring a boat, which has to stand off the island while the vet does what is necessary. This can cost more than the value of a beast in calf, so they sometimes have to shoot the animal. When I understood the question, the answer was still no!

The swan is exhausted and is in no hurry to move away from me. It is, however, making it quite clear that it's not dead yet and will have a go at me if I get too close. Stan, meanwhile, is assisting me from two hundred yards away, just in case the bird decides to make a run for it. I suppose he wants a head start. I've done this before, though, with our geese, so armed with another of those large grey blankets I saved from the flitting, I approach from behind. Giving the bird no time to think, the blanket is thrown over its head and wings before I unceremoniously pounce on it. Once you've got the wings pinned and the feet held firmly, they stop struggling. It's best to carry them backwards though, that way they can't get at your face with their beak. This swan hasn't any energy to struggle and is really quite light under my arm. I guess it's not been able to eat well enough for a while.

Stan is happy for me to ride in the back of the van. He's distinctly unhappy with the look of the bird at close range, even when I keep it wrapped in the blanket. Once we're back at the house, I bed the bird down in the little wooden shed. The swan still looks magnificent up close, its snow-white feathers contrasting with the red of its long beak. It's very weak, though, and has been unwell for a while. There's not much more I can do for it tonight other than allow it to rest safe from the wind. I'll make some phone calls in the morning.

All the boys have seen the swan now, although we're careful not to disturb it too much. I like them to be involved in the care of wild animals. I hope it teaches them about compassion as well as letting them experience the cycle of life. They have loads of questions as usual but the hardest is always from Peedie. 'Will it die, Daddy?'

It did. Overnight, in the warm box of straw, its head

sank slowly down and rested on the rough bedding surrounding and protecting it from the elements. Did it sing before it died? I doubt it; the energy for singing had long gone. The loss of vitality at the point of death always affects me. As if I'm looking at a shell plucked from the tide margin, devoid of its occupant, leaving no suggestion of the delicate life it once nurtured. Only an outline remains, a pencil drawing that time will erase as the shell mingles with the rest of the sand and only the memory lingers.

I'm sad we weren't able to do the simple things for Ivan the way we could for the swan. We couldn't bring him to a sheltered place for his last moments as a massive heart attack took hold; nobody could. We didn't know. Being alone, not lonely but alone, is part of living in these remote places. It can be comforting to let the place surround you and put things in perspective. To allow the isolation, the protection from intrusion, to clear your mind and let you see the world differently. Being alone at the point of death is different, though, I'm less sure about that. No one should die alone if it can be avoided.

Birth

I am Eid-ey,
The isthmus isle, the connector of tidal lands.

I too have borne.

My Calf
by Viking lords so named,
Separated from me slowly.
Peeled away in the flood of the inescapable sea.

A river of time and tide
Flowing through the Sound.
Breaking my grasp
and
Holding her beyond my reach.
She shelters still,
Alone,
Cradled in my head.

Now this woman
Must hold her newborn fast
or
Suffer
My pain of perpetual separation.

14

To Sing or Cry

Eventually, the long weeks of separation are reaching an end. Our school-age boys have permission to skip school for two weeks, homework has been allocated, holiday houses on the mainland booked (we needed two houses as we couldn't get one for the whole fortnight), flights to Aberdeen arranged. The whole house is excited, with its new white exterior, freshly painted staircase, glossy varnished wood front door and bouncing children. It is also being cleaned even more furiously by Nana as she worries more about the birth. We can't leave until Saturday, when Trevor the locum arrives from Exeter in Devon on the morning flight. We're tied to the island until then; breaking free requires planning. All our holiday packing has to be loaded into the van by Wednesday to be sent to Kirkwall as cargo. We'll follow it on Saturday afternoon. I've had to hire the *Guide*, a little passenger boat, to make a special trip to collect us. The whole exercise has taken on the quality of an expedition and that's only to get us to Kirkwall.

People, tractors, vans crowd around the old stone pier, the island parliament, while the sun's sharp rays glitter on the waves under the approaching MV *Islander*. The large dent on her bow is picked out in the bright, reflected sunlight, rusting where the heavy metal plate has creased, cracking the black paint. She's an old boat, strong, tough as an Orcadian boat should be, able to sail in all weathers. Today's summer sun is unflattering; she looks her best in a winter gale, proudly thumping her way through a smoking sea. The hard work of delivering goods to all the North Isles, from cut flowers to bags of cement, falls to her. Manoeuvring at close quarters is an art form as she has no bow thrusters to push her head round. Tides have to be right before she can dock, and those tides dictate the timing of her visits to each North Isle. Ropes are thrown and secured as she hauls herself round against the pier, engines fully astern to avoid being drawn on to the island and hitting the pier nose with her bow again.

The first of three forward hatches is drawn back and the little derrick drops four chains with hooks into the blackness, returning with a half-size metal ship's container, spinning, swinging to and fro, before being landed on the uneven stone pier. A second container is drawn up and deposited beside the first. The only cargo to be loaded is our VW van, so the little derrick drops into the empty hold and comes up again, like one of those dipping novelty birds you used to see in gift shops. The next second, the van is raised high into the air, swinging wildly, repeating its nodding dog impersonation that alarmed me all those months ago. It spins over the side of the boat and at exactly the correct point of rotation plummets into the waiting hold once more. Stage one is complete.

The chaos of the previous few days dies down now the van is away. No more chasing the boys to decide what they want to take on holidays, saving of clothes, cramming as much as possible into the van. Food has been topped up for the ducks and geese, which Trevor is happy to feed when he does surgeries. Trevor will stay as usual with the Traills at the north end beside Calf Sound, so the house doesn't need to be especially tidy. Nana inevitably thinks otherwise, though, and, despite being told not to, has been hanging upside down out the kitchen windows in a form of extreme cleaning I've not seen before. The boys are restless, unsettled and in a hurry to see Mummy again. They're going on a holiday to get a new baby. If only it were that simple.

'When will we get the new baby?'

'It can sit on my hor'sh!'

'Is it a boy or a girl?'

'Will it be wrinkly and pee a lot when it comes, like Matthew did?'

Will 'it' come at all? *If it comes.* That thought, the anxiety still present every time someone mentions the arrival date.

'It will be bright pink with green spots and orange hair,' I say, biting my tongue and pulling on a smile.

'Aw! Dad, be serious!'

I was.

Friday night, and Nana can't stand or sit without being sick. Lying down is all she can manage and only if she doesn't move her head at all. Extreme cleaning has brought on an attack of vertigo and she is now under strict orders to rest which, given her inability to move, she may just follow. I've given her tablets to ease things while we consider if we can travel tomorrow.

The morning is grey and cold as we all pile into Freya's taxis for the trip to the pier, Nana moving very slowly, staggering against me as she's helped into the front seat. She had a large injection of sedative an hour ago to ease the swirling nausea. For a long time, it has felt as if this day would never come, the day of escape, the start of coming together again.

Unlike the day Nana arrived on the island, with its bright cheerful sunshine, the island is dismal today. Grey clouds low in the sky, a restless, mist-covered choppy sea splashes us as we carefully climb down the glistening stone steps to the boat. Martin and Matthew clamber over the gunwale, kicking bits of flaking green paint into the water, dashing into the cabin, as I lift a wriggling Peedie over the side, followed by an enigmatic Mikey, unfazed by the new experience. Nana is lying on her own in the lower cabin, half-dozing, hoping the swell will not be so marked down there.

As the ropes are cast off, I finally break free from the island after months of continuous responsibility. Long months of waiting by the phone, dealing with everything, threadworm, nits, chickenpox, heart attacks and ulcers. Those nine months were easy compared to the weeks of separation, of waiting on another type of phone call, being on the other side, being a relative.

Sailing far out beyond the headland, we pass the lonely figure standing up in a tiny rowing boat. A man held on the water surface, currents ebbing and flowing around him as he hauls his creels. In control and vulnerable simultaneously. Slowly he disappears beyond the horizon as the skipper swings the boat's head round into the waves and she punches her way south, away from Eday to Kirkwall.

In contrast to the sail from Eday to Kirkwall, the journey further south becomes hectic, rushed, as I am swept up in a new sea of people needing to be somewhere. After leaving the boys with Nana, travelling on my own to Aberdeen starts quietly enough, with Kirkwall Airport relaxed and polite. Most of the passengers are obviously heading south to work again, practised in the routines of the flight and indifferent to the safety talks. I haven't flown in a large plane before – I've never needed to.

In Kirkwall, out on the runway, I am fascinated as the plane engines come up to full revs and I feel the aircraft tugging against her own brakes, wanting to be free to fly. The release of the stored energy pushes me back into my seat, the acceleration more than I've ever felt before and I love it. Driving at speed is exciting but this is completely different. Briefly I forget why I am going south, losing myself in the flight. As we break through the thick low cloud, it has never occurred to me that the cloud tops would be white. All the physics I had learned on light refraction and reflection haven't prepared me for the ocean of tumbling vapour folding and unfolding around me. Up in the sky I am briefly free from the world. I can choose to go where I want – in my mind at least. Something that hasn't been possible for a long time.

Landing is less exciting, the thump down on to the tarmac beginning a process of rushing and pushing that I have forgotten about in the nine months since we left Glasgow. It is an overused comparison but people really do behave like sheep, rushing forwards with the herd, only to mill about in bleating dissatisfaction when they get to the next locked gate. I am deliberately last off the plane and immediately disorientated by the noise and the lights of the airport concourse. Signs with arrows, lists of places – departure lounges, arrivals, gates, check-ins. Eventually I make my way to a taxi rank and hide in the back of a cab while the city screams by.

Arriving at the entrance to Aberdeen Maternity Hospital and stepping out of the car, I hesitate to go in. Instead, I walk across to a little grassy area surrounded by trees. Looking high up, the sky is still in place but the land has shrunk, drawn back into little islands of green, defended temporarily from the assault of buildings by rows of metal railings. It isn't going to be easy to feel any rhythm here, the ebb and flow of nature beaten down, drowned under human and mechanical noise.

Once I find my way to the Orkney rooms – the accommodation for relatives provided by the Island's Council above the maternity suite – I trail back down the stairs in search of the antenatal ward. The 'before-birth' ward. A title that rolls up a whole series of emotions into two words held together by an umbilical cord. Maggie has had rough 'before-birth' times in the past, fracturing her ribs from coughing so much with newly diagnosed and uncontrolled asthma during our first pregnancy. At least then I could help out as much as possible. This time I've been able to do nothing for her but send trivia in letters and have stilted telephone conversations, all the while begging the antenatal umbilical cord to stay in place and not rupture.

Now, finally pushing open the door to Maggie's room and slipping quietly round it, she doesn't hear me come in. I want to look at her just for a moment before she sees me and reaffirm the bond that was remade when we moved to Eday. To reconnect the line between us that was ruptured when the plane fought its way into the April skies, buffeted by the north wind, and took her away. I hardly dare to breathe as I watch her sitting beside the bed, working intently on a long-stitch tapestry. The cream threads weave back and forwards across her knee as she finishes the picture of a tawny owl she told me about on the phone. Careful, precise actions placing each thread as accurately as she can to create a gift for me when I arrive. Why would I need a gift?

Eventually, she looks up and smiles without any sign of surprise, knowing that I was there all the time. A gentle smile flickers briefly and then vanishes. We've been apart too long. In self-protection she has shut herself down, turned inwards to survive the long wait, remote and alone. As I reach for her hand in our light fingertip touch her eyes say everything that is needed. The corners of each eye crinkle just a little in pleasure as her relief at my arrival registers in the greens and blues. Carelessness would make me miss how much she loves me.

As I unpack a huge envelope of pictures and cards that the boys have made for their mum, my eye catches sight of the one Matthew made weeks ago stuck proudly to the wall beside her bed. She has a bundle of other cards and letters too, all carefully preserved to take home. Nothing is ever discarded. The rest of our afternoon is taken up with stories, filling in the details missing from the letters I sent. Days on the peat banks cutting and drying the thick black peat, Peedie's potty-training and Nana's exasperation and final pride when he cracked it. She left the proceeds in the potty to show me when I came home – dear knows why! I was spared this, however, as the dog ate them. He was prone to that. It's not the first time he's eaten the baby's nappy sponge, leaving us mystified as to where it has gone. Until the next day, that is, when a yellow or blue foam poo appeared in the garden. Gradually, Maggie and I settle back into our routine. Seriousness and laughter mix freely until evening, and the time for me to go upstairs to my room.

The next morning, waking in the Orkney rooms I hear the shore song of the birds again. At least in my half-stupor I think I do. This time, though, it's nesting gulls on the roof of the maternity suite. Their call is harsh, rasping against my ears and irritating me awake. The sound has none of the melody of the mingling voices of peewits and oystercatchers searching the shoreline for food, reassuring me that all is well. Here, the island's nightwatchman's call has been replaced by the harsh squabbling reality of the city. The gulls have rough nests of sticks and city rubbish scattered unevenly across the flat roof below my window.

Each pair defending the area they have marked out from intruders, shouting and squabbling with neighbours over perceived threats and intrusions. There's none of the cooperative approach of the oystercatchers feeding together in the tangle of sea-washed weed. The seashore browsers maintain a polite distance between themselves but each bird remains alert for a threat to the flock, the whole group sticking together. Here, it's everyone for themselves.

A gull leaves her nest of sticks briefly to fend off a neighbour wandering too close. As soon as the white of her eggs is visible another bird dives on the nest to seize one. The scream from the mother is human, a high-pitched howl of anguish from a young girl in extreme distress as she flies at the murderer. They twist and weave through the sky until the killer callously drops the egg on the grass below to save himself from the pursuit. The mother somersaults in the air and swoops back to the rooftop, where her mate has only just managed to defend the remaining clutch. There's a precariousness to life here, a randomness, a self-inflicted viciousness that isn't apparent on the island. There, the wind sets the cycle of life and to survive you need to cooperate, to tolerate your neighbours without spite. Today, Maggie and I need to work together to ensure the birth of our next child.

Although I'm familiar with the hospital environment – one where I can see the pathways, the tracks weaving through the day – I'm not comfortable. I feel alien, unsure what to do. Back in Maggie's room just after breakfast, I'm uncomfortable in the role of a relative. Disabled and limited in freedom. Even picking up the chart at the end of the bed seems to be frowned upon, as the midwife fixes me with a look of distrust. She takes the chart from me in a pretence of recording some new number. I pick it up again as soon as she lays it down.

I'm used to moving freely in a medical setting. Going in and out of rooms – always with care to knock first. When I did my GP training my senior trainer, a very experienced east end of Glasgow man, told me always to knock before entering a bedroom. 'It gives them time to stop what they're doing,' he would say with a knowing smile. Dear knows what he saw before he started knocking. Today, I can't move about and ask questions. Reading case notes isn't allowed. Even walking out into the corridor in search of a toilet seems like an intrusion, with quizzical looks thrown in my direction. A bit like a wandering gull on the roof, I feel pushed and buffeted until I retreat to our nest in Maggie's room to be with our single egg. Protecting it from any last-minute theft. If it comes.

Anaesthetists come and go. Maggie has an epidural placed in her back. The pain of the manipulated needle squeezing between her vertebrae only registers as a long unwavering look into my eyes. This time I squeeze her hand firmly and hold it for as long as she needs. At last I can do something. Once the epidural is in place the consultant comes in and confirms that Maggie will go to theatre shortly for an internal examination. If he's happy with what he finds he'll rupture her membranes and induce her labour. As he says the words 'rupture her membranes', I'm reminded why I hate obstetrics – it's barbaric. The juxtaposition of words associated with the whole process create a medieval scene.

> **Rupture** – *a severe injury in which an internal part of your body tears or bursts open*
>
> **Membrane** – *a thin pliable sheet of material*

Obstetricians don't speak of gently parting the thin pliable skin protecting the unborn child from the outside world – they rupture it.

> **Induce** – *to persuade or encourage someone to do something*
>
> **Labour** – *to do something with difficulty*

Even when the words appear to be a little softer they're not. Women are not persuaded and encouraged into labour – they have a needle stuck in their arm and chemicals poured in to make the womb contract painfully. I know the science of this process well and I understand the medical necessity but faced with the prospect of these things happening to Maggie, it's the words that upset me. More carefully chosen words would ease the fear.

The fear is real, sitting outside the theatre waiting. This is the moment when we discover whether the placenta – the disc of tissue filled with blood vessels nourishing our baby – has moved sufficiently up and away from the neck of the womb. If it hasn't, the gentle parting of the birth membrane – for that is actually how it's done – will rupture the placenta and blood will pour freely away from Maggie and our baby simultaneously. Through the open door of the theatre, I can see a roomful of people in theatre greens surrounding Maggie. After a few minutes, they simply disperse. Each walking past me and off to some other task. My first thought is that our baby is dead. Nothing more needs to be done. Just as I'm trying to shake this out of my head, the consultant stops in front of me.

'It's fine. We'll progress with labour and she should deliver this afternoon.'

Then he walks away, leaving me once again on my own. Senior medics seem to do that. Make a statement and then walk away without asking if you're okay with the information they've just given you. There's a sense that we should know the detailed ins and outs of any situation because, after all, we're doctors too. Actually, I'm not a doctor today, I'm a relative, with all the hopes and anxieties of any new father-to-be. I want someone to treat me like that and not assume I'm comfortable.

With Maggie moved to the labour ward, we have a room to ourselves again. The large window looks out over the same grassy area I used as a little haven before coming into the hospital yesterday. We're higher up now, with the window safe from prying eyes. We have more space, more light around us, and a sky to watch. Maggie is sitting up in bed, superficially comfortable, but I can see she isn't. Once again, her eyes tell me things others can't see. She's scared. Not just of the birth but of the inevitable pain that will precede it. In all her other deliveries she has never been able to get good pain relief. The usual entonox – a gaseous mixture of nitrous oxide and air – that should reduce pain perception has no effect at all. Pain-killing injections of any type equally don't work. For the moment, though, she hasn't any pain as the drip full of carefully measured doses of syntocinon begins to induce the womb to contract.

As the morning drifts into afternoon, the drip in Maggie's arm is doing its work as the contractions steadily increase into full labour. We're mostly silent now, watching clouds scud across the skies and the leaves sway in the gentle wind blowing through the trees around the little park. As she dozes, I begin to believe we will have a new baby. The baby's heart monitor is beeping away steadily, hardly wavering with each contraction. In previous pregnancies, I've had to turn the sound off on the machine and face it away from Maggie as she became anxious about the rapid slowing of the baby's heart with each contraction. She would feel it was her failure to labour properly that made our baby distressed. We would almost hold our breath as we waited for the heart rate to slowly creep back up to normal. The longer it took, the more stress our baby was under. This time there's nothing to worry either of us. Maggie is peaceful and feeling no pain at all now the epidural is working.

About three o'clock I burst out laughing so loudly a midwife looks round the door.

'What's the matter?'

'She has a slight headache,' I say, to the annoyance of the midwife, who clearly disapproves of my lack of sympathy.

'Would you like something for it, Mrs Alexander?' she asks, looking severely at me all the time.

'No, I'm okay, it's nothing.'

As the midwife leaves the room again, Maggie fixes me with a stare, raising one eyebrow as she does it.

'What's so funny about my headache? I have a slight ache in the front of my head.'

'I know, but after all the anxiety and worry since you bled I've been dreading today and what might happen. And the worst thing that has happened is you have a slight headache.'

She reaches out and gives my hand a gentle squeeze.

It's the last gentle squeeze of the day, however, as it

seems the slight headache was the start of the second stage of labour. The room fills with people and equipment again. We begin our practised routine of delivery. Not one we've learned from any antenatal classes, but our own one, built from experience. Now I only give Maggie my first two fingers to hold on to and crush as the epidural is allowed to wear off. As a junior father during Martin's birth, I gave her my whole hand as the effort of pushing began. It was two days before my hand worked properly again. A small sacrifice, I know, but nevertheless.

There's only one person in the press of people in the room who reassures me just by being there. Still unjustly regarding the whole practice of obstetrics as medieval, it is the sight of the young paediatrician that settles my nerves. I know her role and understand the equipment she has with her. Once we have our baby out in the open, we can sort any problem out. So long as it's still inside, enclosed in the remnants of the ruptured egg sac, the obstetric machine prevents us caring for it. Even as a junior paediatrician, I hated the waiting for the baby to arrive, feeling nothing but nerves. Once I was handed the tiny bundle of towels and mucus, I was fine. No matter what the colour the tiny scrap was or how lifeless it seemed, I knew what to do next. So, today I reassure myself by looking over and seeing myself standing at the back of a crowd of people waiting for another baby.

Without any further fuss she's here. Our first daughter

has her face wiped with towels and the little bundle is held up for us to see before being handed to the paediatrician. I don't feel anything at first, as I'm still clinically appraising everything in the room. Maggie seems fine, the baby wasn't blue and floppy, the consultant isn't worried, the nurses aren't fidgeting with equipment. Everything is as it should be. Only after my assessment is complete can I allow myself to feel things again.

'What a proud dad you'll be with a daughter.'

'You'll be so glad it's not another son, how many have you already?'

'Oh, a little girl, wonderful ...'

'She's beautiful, you'll be spoiling her ...'

The irritating gender-biased voices wash over me, as all I feel is relief. Maggie is alive and our baby is alive and, well, that is enough for now. Recovering a little after all the effort, Maggie asks for a tissue from her handbag in the locker beside her bed. Rummaging in the worn soft leather bag, the only one she has, I shove aside the two screwdrivers, a set of pliers, some wool and a crochet hook before I can see the packet at the bottom of the bag. The tools are legacies from her anaesthetic days, when she had to adjust the gas machines herself. One screwdriver, the flat-headed one, taken from her sewing machine box, has the word SINGER stamped on it.

It's as well Maggie is tough, as this pregnancy isn't over yet. The placenta is fused to the side wall of her womb by the bleeding weeks earlier. The damaged area is fibrous and adherent, which is probably the reason there was no further haemorrhage, but it also means she has to endure the pain of its removal. A final twist for her after six weeks of worrying the placenta would sheer away. Now each piece has to be picked off by hand to ensure there is no place for infection to take hold. The consultant looks up from his task, his face mask shoved up on his forehead.

'Who would do this for a living?' he says.

I've had enough of obstetrics and, once Maggie is settled again, I decide to go outside for a few moments. Once I'm here in the fresh air, I can breathe again. I walk slowly around the little park with a contented smile on my face, looking up into the trees and sky, using them to take me away from the city. The gulls still circle overhead but they're mostly quiet now in the late afternoon. Further over, away from the main entrance, there's a group of bushes, nothing special, just those thick green bushes you see in parks. In the space between them something white on the ground catches my eye. Turning it over with my foot, the eggshell is quite fresh but smashed on one side by a powerful beak. Standing looking at the destroyed dream beside my foot, my thoughts return to the phone call all those weeks ago. To the chaos in my head immediately afterwards, the uncontrolled fear. Finally, to the peat fire burning in a grate as the grey mist of the evening's rain was parted by the island sunlight briefly entering the room. Be still and know that I am God.

Megan. The first letter of her name would always have to be an 'M'. Martin, Matthew, Michael, Murray and Megan. None of that was intentional until we got to Michael and someone said his name would have to be 'M' as well. So now we are seven Ms, and all totally different people. The tiniest of us is now learning her first lesson – breastfeeding. She seems to be doing pretty well too, cuddled up under the blue cellular blanket that all hospitals seem to have. Around 8 p.m. the room door opens and the consultant appears again, this time without his face mask.

'How's everything? You can relax now,' he says, then he turns to Sister. 'Anything to worry us? No! Good, you can get home in the morning if everything stays the same overnight. I won't see you again until the next one.' Turning to speak to me, he says, 'Malcolm, I've made you medical escort for your wife, otherwise we couldn't get clearance to fly her back so soon. You'll be fine with that, won't you?' And with that, he rescinds my status as relative.

The next morning the 'waiting bag' which was packed all those weeks earlier and placed in the locker of the little plane is carefully repacked. This time minus a tiny white baby jacket with pearlized buttons, a satin-ribbon-trimmed bonnet and a pair of bootees. The tiny glint of optimism all those weeks ago proving correct as Megan lies in my arms, unaffected by the activity around her. Soon we're in the departure lounge at the airport, surrounded by knowing looks and smiles as we wait on the flight back to Kirkwall. Before long, we're ushered on to the plane and shown to our seats. Maggie is given a separate lap strap for Megan, who has to be secured to her mum for take-off. The strap is huge as it wraps round our little bundle and doesn't really look as though it will do anything other than tip her upside down if we stop quickly.

Neither the feeling of acceleration nor the noise of take-off seems to upset Megan as she dozes on her mum's lap. As I look across at them both and out of the window, once again we're back above the clouds in the realm of freedom. The cloud is more broken today and we can see the sea below as we travel north. Maggie is quiet, gazing out as the world slowly passes beneath her, lost in her own thoughts. Looking down again at my daughter, wrapped in her oversized protective seatbelt, the stupidity of it makes me shake my head.

'Why are you shaking your head?' asks Maggie. 'Are you okay?'

'Just thinking.'

'About ...?'

'How pointless that seatbelt is wrapped round Megan. We needed it weeks ago to hold her inside you, not now to hold on to her outside you. We're not going to let her go now we've got her.'

15

Now She's Come

For the second week of Maggie's recuperation, we moved from a holiday cottage to a working farm called Cornquoy. The place is surrounded by everything the boys love. Fields, animals and sea. The cottage in the farmyard is an old farm labourer's cottage, reminding me of ones I saw as a boy playing on the farms around the village. We quickly settle into the routine of a new baby with plenty of extra hands to help at the moment. Maggie's mum is feeling better now she has stopped trying to clean everything in sight and is totally focussed on the new baby. The boys' initial fascination with their tiny sister is beginning to wane. Peedie is disappointed, as she isn't bright pink with green spots and orange hair. He's particularly surprised to find she doesn't have a willy either.

When Maggie is breastfeeding, I have always felt fairly redundant in a baby's life. Not unnecessary, as there's still plenty of things to do, like nappy changes and such like, but I'm not really fulfilling my role as Dad for our new arrival. I'm even more superfluous today, as Nana is intent on holding Megan as soon as she's finished feeding. I don't mind, as other than a feeling of fascination at the tiny life we have been given to look after, I've never felt much else when our babies have been this small. I much prefer it when we can start to communicate with smiles and those daft sounds all fathers make to amuse babies. In a little while no doubt, I'll pretend to blow out the electric lights by magic and make toy animals mysteriously appear and disappear. Bedtime stories will follow on eventually but for now I'm redundant – or I would be if we didn't have four other children.

We've taken a football and the red Frisbee out into the field beside the cottage but there's no chance of playing with them as the boys are distracted by the 'caddie' lambs. The farmer's wife has come out with bottles of milk for the orphans – the lambs, not our boys, who just look like orphans – and immediately Matthew is straight across to help. What follows looks for all the world like a mini tug of war as the lambs fix firmly to the rubber teat and draw the bottle towards them. Several times Peedie, who is determined to do the same as his brothers, lets out a little squeak and leaps backwards as the lamb pulls the bottle away from him. There are eggs to be gathered too, from the shed at the end of our cottage. Fresh brown eggs, still with the feeling of warmth from the hen and the sweet musty smell of straw. Unfortunately, we can't eat them as both Martin and Michael are acutely allergic to them. The eggs are carefully placed in a small pail and given to the farmer's wife.

'Come on, boys, we'll go for a walk,' I shout once the feeding and gathering is done. 'We'll leave Mum and Nana to get some peace.'

'Can we bring the Frisbee?'

'Bring what you like. Go and get your jackets, it's a bit windy.'

The Frisbee flies back and forth between us, hovering above Peedie's head and making him spin around in circles before falling over. Sometimes the wind tugs it away unexpectedly and there's a mad scrambling and chasing to catch it. Martin loves to throw himself into the heather to grab it, rolling over and over in springy turf, and flattening the tall grasses singing in the wind. Perhaps Mike is less involved in the game, as he looks in the ditches and pulls up the long strands of grass to use as tickling devices. As we wander on down the track it's clear all of us are at home in this land of grass and wind.

The wind grabs the Frisbee and throws it once more over a battered wire fence, the wire squeaking and squealing as I climb over to retrieve it. The ground is undulating and there appears to be a circle lying under the turf, hidden by years of growth. A tiny plaque buried deep in the heather says this is one of the few disc barrows in Britain. A protective circle shaped around the rectangular barrow. These sites have been thought to be burial sites of important women in the Stone Age. There have been people living and working on this land for over 2,500 years. Children running, falling, shouting, laughing, just like we are. All in a continuous flow of time.

'Boys, come here ... listen.'

'What we listening for, Dad?'

'Nothing ... just listen ...'

They're used to me doing this now. Making them stop and look or listen or both. I don't know if they'll do this when they grow up but I want to try to teach them to step off the world just for a minute. To simply be alive in a landscape. By stopping, I would often see things I would have missed. Perhaps a shy treecreeper quietly spiralling up the trunk of an oak tree, searching for bugs hidden in the bark, or a stoat standing erect, looking and listening like me. Other times, I would study the way a single leaf shivers and shakes on a tree of motionless leaves in a summer calm. As if the leaf is trying to break free while everyone else is asleep. Maybe more of us should try to break free too.

'I'sh can't hear anything ... just wind.'

'I know ... wind shaking the heather. What does it sound like?'

A pause as they listen again ...

'Like the telly when it doesn't work ... all staticky and hissy ... when the signal gets broken.'

'Mmm ... good description, Martin. It sounds like sand to me, blowing along the beach. Do you know there have been people living on this very spot for thousands of years? Listening to the very same sounds of the wind.'

Another silence.

'Dad, the Frisbee's gone over the fence again!'

We turn round and tumble and laugh our way back to the cottage as the moment created by the wind is broken by it, too.

It's here I must break my story and tell you that even now, almost thirty years later, I don't understand what happened next when we returned to the cottage. On one or two occasions only I have had a strange dream that I remember when I'm awake. Dreaming is not unusual for me but the dreams I'm thinking about are not the absurd nonsense that can be tracked back to events of the previous few days – those odd dreams we have when events become a soup of happenings that our brains are trying to process and file. Nor do I mean the dream I came to recognize as happening at times of stress, when I was responsible for something that wasn't working out as it should. In those dreams, which were more regular as I became senior in the Health Service, I would be responsible for large cats which were roaming free and hungry. Tigers were most common, hunting across countryside that was solely in my charge. Eventually, I learned to wake myself from that dream, identifying it for what it was. The very few occasions I'm thinking about are nothing like any other dreams I have had. Let me continue my story.

Once we are back at the cottage, it is definitely time for a drink and biscuits. Our favourites are Jammie Dodgers, those bright iced rings with red sticky jam in the middle. Wellies and jackets are peeled off and hung around the doorway while the boys gather round Megan to chat to her. Matthew tells her about the Frisbee and the wind, a story which makes no impression on her at all as she sleeps in Maggie's arms, while I go in search of the juice and biscuits in the little kitchen at the back of the cottage. It would perhaps be better described as a kitchenette with a stainless-steel sink below the window, old-fashioned wooden cupboards painted cream hung on one wall and a gas cooker on the other. The wallpaper is cream and decorated with little red hearts, making the room feel like a child's playroom rather than a kitchen. I can't find the biscuits. Nothing unusual, as I regularly can't find things Maggie has put away.

'Where did you put the biscuits, love?'

'Hang on, I'll get them. Put the kettle on too, will you? I need a coffee.' I've just filled the kettle and put it on the cooker when she walks into the room.

'Take the baby, will you, and I'll find the biscuits.'

Taking her in my arms, I gently fold the outsized dress Nana bought in Kirkwall around her. The smallest dress the shop had. She lies peacefully, my daughter, snuggled down in the crook of my arm as I relax again now we are all together. As I raise my head to look out the kitchen window to the fields beyond, everything around me appears to stop, as if the flow of time has hesitated, failing to move forwards for just an instant. I've been in this moment before. Then, it was a ludicrous dream I had when we stayed in Glasgow not long after Murray was born two years ago. Now, it is real and around me. Ludicrous because of the setting. In my dream, I was holding a new baby girl in a room of a small house which we lived in. The room was this one. Window, sink, cupboards, cooker and the ludicrous part – the wallpaper with red hearts all over. I remember waking from that dream all those years before and thinking, *That will never happen.* We would never have a house with red heart wallpaper and certainly not more children, we're not even speaking to each other!

The moment was brief but it remains unsettling to this day. I have no explanation for how such dreams come about. I am certain they are remembered dreams separated in time from the later event, and not the oddity that is déjà vu, which is explained by an interruption in the process of making memories where a current event is played back almost instantly in your head as a memory, making you think you've been there before. Does island life make you more susceptible, more open, to these happenings?

Tonight, I've lit the open fire in the sitting room and played a few games with the boys. My story about Angus Seagull – one of many I've made up over the years – has drawn to a close, so it's time for bed. Megan has been restless tonight, not quite settled yet into a good feeding pattern. It often happens a few days after the birth, before Maggie's milk supply comes in properly. The only one who has been able to get her to relax is Matthew. He sat through all the games and stories propped up in the old armchair by the fire with his legs straight out in front of him and his arms wrapped firmly round Megan's middle. Now the fire is dying back and the flicker of red flames plays across his sleepy face. He still refuses to go to sleep.

'Time for bed, Matthew, give Megan to me now ...'

'No,' he says as his eyes fall closed again. 'She's my sister.'

'I know, pal, and she'll be your sister in the morning too ... now she's come.'

16

Heart Stop

I've developed an addiction for flakey biscuits from the Westray baker, so before we sail back to the island it's time for a raid on the Kirkwall shops. There are two choices for our attack. Cummings and Spence, a general store, and the eponymously named Frozen Food shop, both in Albert Street. Like many pirates on raiding trips, after completing our first attack on the general store we find we aren't satiated so both locations are invaded by five wide-eyed boys with money to spend. Having pocket money is a new phenomenon for our gang. There is no point in allocating weekly sums of money on the island, where there is nowhere to spend it. Instead, we have generous holiday money to feed the desires of sweet-munching pirates. Chupa Chups lollies are one of the favourites of the moment. Brightly coloured spheres of sugar, just waiting to be sucked with a satisfying slurp at the end of each 'chupa'.

After a day of raiding and skirmishing around Kirkwall, the van is now packed again with supplies for the coming summer and parked once more on the pier. We're all staying with Mrs Stevenson in Dundas Crescent tonight, the boys occupying the huge bay-windowed bedroom that overlooks the garden. We stayed here on our way out to Eday all those months ago and it's relaxing being back with this kind lady, who treats the boys as her own. Her delight at seeing Megan is maternal as she carefully takes the 'peedie lass' from Maggie and through into the sitting room. The house itself is plainly furnished but feels homely. The atmosphere, the comfort, is entirely down to Mrs Stevenson's attitude which, like many folk in the isles, is entirely welcoming and without prejudice. Folks are who they are and it's not for others to judge.

In the evening, there's time for me to take a walk round town on my own. Unlike the cities south, the town is peaceful as the simmer dim, that nightly long spell of almost daylight, lights the north side of the copper spire on the cathedral. The reds and yellows of the ancient stone walls are more intense in the searching fingers of low sunlight. Much of the sandstone for the original building came from Eday, quarried along the West Side Road near where Ken grazes his sheep. Stone that was laid down millennia ago when Orkney was formed in the silt of Lake Orcadie. The sandstone now visible in the wind- and salt-weathered walls first compressed into layers of mud and then to soft stone, all the tiny grains of silt drawn down from the Devonian Great North river feeding the lake forced into cooperation to form a solid and lasting rock.

Time always seems to be visible on the surface of the land in Orkney. No matter where you are, the line of it breaks through the soil, the indelible imprint of geology and man captured side by side. Whether it is rock stacks or neolithic standing stones, deep sea-cut geos or Viking boat knousts, Devonian sandstone on the face of the cathedral – the millennia break through, touching centuries, minutes and seconds. You can't help but see an ordinary day's events in the context of time. Nothing is ever just an event or an incident. There isn't an illness or disease. Each is part of something continuous, more meaningful. Perhaps I began to understand this when I read Nessie's medical card all those months ago and saw her life set out concisely on the surface of the Lloyd George envelope. Standing now in front of the cathedral in the near midnight sun, I'm aware that my education is only just beginning.

The next morning we're all back on Eday, met by Claire at the pier who helps ferry us up to the house. I phoned Claire when Megan was born so everyone knows about the new arrival. There's a steady stream of visitors to the house, with various gifts and mindings for the wee one. Plans are soon in place for her christening in six weeks' time, with Maggie deciding to host an open house afterwards for the whole island. Nana will stay until the christening is over and then return home to the Isle of Bute to recover.

A week later and two presents arrive at our door. The first is a sizeable box delivered by Stan on his way back from the airstrip. Lifting it quickly into the surgery, I'm keen to ensure the contents are in one piece. I cut the securing tape and discard the outer box, revealing a LIFEPAK 10. The ultimate in out-of-hospital care heart monitors. A portable ECG and defibrillator with external pacing capability. Not only that, it comes in a bright-red case. As I look at it, I can feel myself relaxing a little more. Now I have enough equipment to give most people a fighting chance until the air ambulance can get here. With this magnificent machine not only can I monitor heart rhythms but I can correct some with shock therapy. For others, I can take over the rhythm and provide the electrical stimulus externally through the chest wall. This is the most up-to-date piece of kit around and I've only got it because of my time on Health Board committees when we were south. At the end of each financial year, the Boards have sums of money left over that come under the category of use it or lose it. If you know when to ask, you stand a chance of getting new equipment, so I placed my request in February to the Chief Medical Officer. Not everything up here is about wind and weather. Everything is about timing, though.

'Maggie, come and see this machine,' I holler through to the kitchen. 'It's amazing.'

'Is that the defib here now? I hope it's worth all that money.'

'Of course it is, look at what it can do.'

'It had better make tea as well. Wasn't it nearly two thousand pounds?'

Ex-anaesthetists can be difficult to please. As a group of clinicians, they're not impressed by fancy machinery, regarding it as a liability and bound to go wrong at the least helpful time. I'm used to this attitude and prattle on excitedly.

'I'll need to set up CPR training for the island now. There's no sense in having a machine like this if no one has kept them breathing until I get there. I think the company rep said she'd come up to see us to make sure everything was working fine. Maybe I'll do them then ...'

'Why are you so excited about this?' she cuts in.

'Because we're safe now. As safe as we can be. We could, if we needed to, ventilate someone for a few hours and monitor their heart. So long as they aren't bleeding to death we can give them a chance.'

'Do you want a coffee?' says the unimpressed one.

'Okay. I'll read the manual while I have one then I can come back and have a play around with it.'

'Go and give the goats some hay and I'll put the kettle on,' she says, dismissing me to the field outside to calm down. Clearly, she regards me as over-optimistic in my assessment of what we could achieve.

As I open our front door, now magnificently coated in a rich deep-brown yacht varnish, I see there's a bag hanging on the handle. There often is nowadays, as folk who don't have the change available for the prescription charge leave equivalent goods instead.

'There are two cabbages on the door handle.'

'Who are they from?'

'No idea, nobody is due to make any payment just now,' I say as I place the Co-op bag on the table. 'I didn't hear anyone at the door.'

'I didn't see cars either when you were playing with your new toy. Only Willick's little blue Mini Metro going over the hill towards Cusebay.'

'Ah, that explains it. The Laird's garden is two cabbages less.'

Later that morning after a phone call to Diane, the company rep for the ECG machine, I take a notice up to the Co-op and pin it on the board. I don't know why I bother to do this, as I just have to tell one person about the plans for CPR sessions and everyone will know. Anyway, we'll fit them in before the school closes. I want to focus the sessions on the women and children of the island. The men are the vulnerable ones here, many of them with blood pressure and cholesterol problems. I often wonder if the diet is wrong now for the way of working. In the past, much of the work would be done by hand-digging and lifting with spade and fork. Now, machines assist a huge amount, with JCBs and tractor attachments easing the workload. Much of the work is still very physical but less so than in the past. The diet, however, remains very high in fat and salt. Tatties boiled and fried in animal fat taste just wonderful. I'm not so sure about salt fish, though, which I was offered by Magnus's wife once. As I pin the notice up I quickly scan the other notices. Sports Day is in two weeks, in the final week of school for this year. Activities and sports for all ages ending with a tug of war. The next event isn't until the school goes back in August, when the annual sale of work takes place.

There's a good-sized field behind the school where the Sports Day is held today. The sun is shining but the wind still blows steadily from the sea, bringing with it the smell of new-mown hay from the hillside below. The field has been cut too, and rough lines laid out for the races. The usual serious races are interspersed with the really tricky ones. The three-legged race; the sack race; the wheelbarrow race. Martin and I have been practising for the wheelbarrow race across the grassy area in our walled garden. We can almost make it over to the other side now without falling. This will be my only event, as the other men's one is beyond me. At a safe distance from the crowd there's a group of younger men practising with a pitchfork and a bale of straw. They heft the bale on the fork and swing it backwards and forwards before launching it into the air.

Wandering across to watch, I'm just in time to see the competition start. Murdo, Claire's son-in-law, swings the bale over an eight-foot-high bar without breaking much sweat. When I think about him lifting the wardrobes up the stairs in Heatherlea, I'm not surprised to see the ease with which the bale leaves the fork. Each of the bales will weigh in at around 60lb, perhaps even heavier if the straw has been damp, so despite the teasing from the younger men I'm not even going to pretend to try. One by one the contestants succeed and then fail to clear the bar, the bale crashing back to the ground instead of landing squarely on the waiting tractor trailer. The macho atmosphere is tangible as the equivalent of Olympic weightlifting takes place on Eday Fields. Shouts and roars of encouragement and derision accompany each attempt. Failure is signalled by the pitchfork being thrown to the ground in disgust.

Gradually, each bale slowly disintegrates under the continual thrashing, as the tough orange binder twine slips from the ends and straw spills around the feet of the contestant. At the end of the contest there's only Hughie left throwing the bale. Throughout the afternoon, his bales have flown over the bar with the same ease I would throw salt over my shoulder. The bar has been lifted again.

Ten feet six inches – higher than the tractor cab roof. This time, there's silence in the group of onlookers as Hughie squares up to a new bale. Hefting it once more to get the measure of it, feeling the balance point as he swings it backwards and forwards. Then, when he's happy, he starts the long back swing but the bale strikes the ground and falls from the fork. Laying the bale down, he picks his spot and drives the twin tines hard into the centre of it. Then, without any further ado, he swings the bale backwards, arches his back, driving the fork forwards and upwards as his left hand slides down the length of the shaft. Using both hands he forces the fork into the air. A roar goes up as the bale hesitates then rolls over the bar on to the trailer. As hands move to raise the bar again Hughie signals enough is enough and retires, victorious, into the waiting crowd.

The next day I'm back at the school with a new friend – Resusci Annie – a rather glamorous training manikin that will let me teach emergency resuscitation. She came out on the early flight with Diane. Training for the women of the island begins at 11 a.m. in the school gym hall. I had intended it to be a fairly serious affair, as we try to ensure the safety of the men on the island. That might sound chauvinistic but it's not really. Many of the men, and some of the women too, have had this sort of training as part of the volunteer fire brigade or as coastguard members. The folks who haven't been trained are the other women and they are most likely to be the first on the scene if their husband takes unwell. Maggie and I aren't the only husband and wife partnership on the island; all the other married folk are partners at work too. Shifting sheep and cattle from hill to farm; fencing the land; cutting the peat; working the silage and hay. So here we are with Annie, collapsed on the gym hall floor, and a group of keen but bemused wives listening to Diane and me talk through the process of saving someone's life.

After a little while it's time for the first volunteer to step forward and have a go. Willa doesn't hesitate and crouches beside Annie, ready for action. After checking her patient is actually unconscious and not breathing, she carefully lifts the dummy's jaw upwards and closes its nostrils with the finger and thumb of her right hand. She takes in a huge breath, leans forward and bursts out laughing, followed by the whole class.

'I canna do it. It's too silly.'

'It seems that way, doesn't it, but one day it might not be,' I say. 'Forget we're all here and think of it on the hillside above the farm, up checking the cattle with your husband. He's just said he still doesn't feel great then he's fallen into the heather and stopped breathing. What's next?'

'I canna shout for help, there's no one around.'

'No, you're right, it's all up to you.'

'Right, he's no responding to me. I can't feel him

breathing even after I've houked up his jaw. There's no pulse ...'

Taking a big breath, she carries on exactly as trained. Two big breaths, then fifteen chest compressions. Time and time again, until either someone else arrives or she has to give up. Exhausted and alone on the hill, she will have to deal with the reality of life here. No matter how trained we are, there are times when we only have each other. We make the best of it and have to accept that sometimes that isn't enough.

In the afternoon, we have a short but exciting session with the whole primary school. They're used to me being their teacher now, so the class sits quietly while we explain what the dummy does and how the fancy ECG machine works. The class ranges from five to eleven years old, so we need to be careful how we say things. Like the wives in the morning session, these children may be the only person around if something happens to a family member. They may well be the only person on the hillside with their dad fixing fences or herding sheep. The session concentrates on making sure they get help as fast as they can, but only after we show the littlest ones a new technique I've invented.

Part of the procedure for a cardiac arrest is to thump the patient firmly in the centre of the chest before starting full CPR. Very occasionally, this has been shown to correct the heart's rhythm and restart it. So today, instead of doing the 'precordial thump', as it is known, we teach the smallest children to do the 'precordial jump'. Well, it's a sit really, where I get them to sit down briskly on to the dummy's chest before running for help. Who knows, maybe someone will tell me one day if it worked.

Once the excitement is over, I return the class to their teacher and then drop Diane off at the airstrip for her flight back. It's a glorious day so she should have an excellent view of the islands as she and Resusci Annie head back to Kirkwall. I'm feeling pleased with myself as I roll carefully to a halt outside the house.

'Hi there,' I say to Maggie, as I breeze into the kitchen then stop. 'What's wrong?'

'I nearly blew myself up!'

'What? How?'

'I left the gas on to the grill but the flame must have gone out,' she says, tearfully. 'Then, when I tried to heat a pan of water the grill door blew open and knocked me over.'

'Are you hurt? Did you get burned?'

'No, just my apron ...'

'But are you all right now?'

'Just shaken now ... I was frightened when there was no one here.'

17

Trust

The day of the August sale of work has arrived and the hall attached to the school is jammed with people looking for bargains. Tables are piled high with all sorts of goods, from the universally popular home baking stall – where the only way to buy anything is through the judicious use of elbows and some accidental toe tramping, always with a smile – to the more unusual, old and barely working farm implements stall. Tea and cake are being served at the front of the hall on a little flock of orphaned tables, dressed in cast-me-down tablecloths to cover the imperfections life has dealt them. A carefully placed beer mat props up a previously fractured and shortened leg. A wooden splint supports a blue metal leg with a terminal case of rust. Colour and race are no barrier to joining this lovingly tended family.

My eye is taken by a set of matching cushions resting resplendent in the centre of a soft goods table. Not that we need cushions but somehow you feel they have a story about them. Eileen of The Bu is quick to tell me that this is their last appearance this year. The cushions are on a final warning from Jenny, who naturally controls all aspects of the sale. If they don't sell this year then ... well, it's not exactly clear what. The overstuffed brocade cushions with expensive piped edges have made an appearance every year for the past five years. They're clearly worth a bit of money and don't show any signs of being used, so there's a visceral antipathy to allowing them to become waste.

Waste is not a natural thing on an island; there is always a further use to be made of almost anything, as the many cars scattered round the fields bear witness to. There are car toolstores, car hay feeders, car chicken houses and, frankly, some cars which are cars-that-might-be-useful-in-the-future cars. There are also the still-running-but-not-legal cars, which have the honour of becoming 'field' cars. Most farms have them for joyriding across the fields. Primary-school-age youngsters, boys and girls, learn to drive these quite expertly long before they can drive on the roads legally. Unfortunately, this doesn't prevent regular testosterone-fuelled tragedies on the isles' roads when they turn seventeen years old. The lack of police presence can make it seem like a speeder's paradise and every island has its tale of wasted lives. Not all waste can be avoided, I'm afraid.

After an hour of browsing, we gather the boys and go home again with a small pile of recycled toys and some nicotiana plants I've optimistically selected for myself. I wonder if anyone will notice the incongruity of a doctor's surgery with tobacco plants growing in the little garden outside. There's a sheltered spot behind the dyke surrounding the yard that will do just fine for them. Hopefully, we'll get the benefit of the scent before summer ends. I noticed the cushions were still sitting regally in the centre of an almost empty table as we left the hall. I wonder what will become of them now?

As summer drifts towards autumn, the familiar patterns of surgeries and home visits combine with afternoon walks, evenings of homework and play. Maggie has a knitting machine and now the mechanical zip of the carriage over the needles replaces the sound of slates rippling across the roof. The machine seems to be fickle and, unless you are very particular about how you do things, there are frequent crashes. We've walked down to The Bu this afternoon to speak to Eileen and let Maggie see her more industrial machines. In the field opposite the farm, the harvest is just beginning, with the oats ripe enough to cut and stack. Leaving the ladies to talk about wool, all five boys cross the stubble to watch the old-fashioned binder cut and tie the sheaves in one movement. I've never seen this before. Even as a boy the farmers used combine harvesters to separate grain and straw.

'It'll be the last time you see this, Doc,' says Thorfinn on the tractor. 'We'll switch to combining next year when Dad retires.'

'Watch how this works, boys. The reaping wheel knocks the stalks on to the cutter then they're swept up on to the conveyor belt and the binder part ties them into bundles.'

'It just spits them out the side, Dad, doesn't it?'

'Look over there where they've been gathered, they're building proper stacks.'

Along the edge of the field, three stacks are slowly rising in perfect circles, grain pointing inwards and stalks outwards. A slight downward slope ensures the rain runs to the outside of the stack. One stack is already complete and capped with a heavy net, held down with stones in preparation for the winter gales. I don't think the boys are that interested: it is just a haystack. They've spotted something on the barbed wire on top of the fence.

'Why is this bee stuck on the prong of the wire, Dad? Did the wind blow it there?'

'No, that isn't really possible. It has been put there.'

'Who did that? That's cruel,' says Matthew.

'A bird. A shrike. It's called the butcher bird because it hangs some of its food up on spikes and hooks. That is really its larder you're looking at.'

'I don't think that bee is going anywhere else now, is it, Dad?'

'No, it will have to stay here with us now, won't it?'

After all that has happened in the past year, staying here doesn't feel like being trapped any more. I'm not held unwillingly on the island, unable to fly freely away. Even after all the time Maggie spent in hospital I can recognize now I was in a more difficult trap in Glasgow. Perhaps the sense of moving back in time has helped, taking me back to my childhood in so many ways. Letting me start again. I can see people more easily now, people in a place, people in time. Not episodes of illness, puzzles to solve, but people to help as life turns around them. As we walk round the field the Arctic terns dive over the bay below us, back again from the Weddell Sea for our summer. It is good to see them but I'm not envious any more.

Now the surgery is smartened up and equipped the way we would like it, I have time to continue putting the patient records on to the computer. Afternoons are spent working my way through each Lloyd George envelope and carefully editing the relevant information into a standardized format. Slowly, stories unfold as I read through each record. I'm just getting into the swing of things this afternoon when I hear Maggie shouting to come and help her. She seems to be outside.

Willick had turned up unannounced at the kitchen

door and knocked politely. When Maggie answered he looked down at his Wellington boot and said, 'I think I've cut my foot,' in his matter-of-fact way.

Blood is flowing freely down the steps on to the path from a broad slice across his Wellington boot. A thick clot is forming, which squeezes out from the gash in the boot as we quickly help him across to the surgery door and into the consulting room. As soon as we sit him in a chair and start to remove his boot the adrenalin that has been keeping him going runs out, the colour draining from his face. He takes on a translucency that is more in keeping with the two pints of blood in his Wellington boot as he passes out and slides to the floor.

Quickly putting gloves on, I remove Willick's sock and clean off the wound with copious amounts of saline from an IV bag, while he apparently sleeps peacefully on the surgery lino. Maggie checks his pulse and airway, which are both okay; his blood pressure is low, though. Fortuitously, this gives me what is known as a 'dry field' with no bleeding, and I can easily fully explore the wound. He never moves when I probe beneath the skin and check the tendons and fascia beneath. The glistening silvery layers of tendon lying below the skin shine much brighter and cleaner than I remember from our anatomy classes. It is fifteen years since I've seen the inside of a foot but from memory everything looks intact. The copious bleeding is coming from superficial arteries which I can just make out at the edges of the wound. Whatever he cut himself on fortunately did more damage to his Wellington than his foot. I clamp off the offending arteries, working quickly to try to complete the repair before he comes around again.

Just as we do this, Peedie runs into the surgery and says, 'Meggie is crying and sh'ish won't stop!'

'Pull her baby bouncer through into the dining room and Mum will be there in a minute.'

'Me an' my hor'sh will do it!'

And he gallops off, with only a passing glance at the unconscious Willick on the floor.

Tying off the superficial arteries beneath the skin, I'm then able to close the single linear wound easily. The lack of local anaesthetic is helpful. Using it causes swelling in the tissues, making the wound line boggy and uneven. This cut is flush and clean, coming together perfectly. Just as the last suture is placed, Willick begins to come around, gazing mystified at the ceiling.

Once we sort out a tetanus booster and antibiotic cover he is much more like himself and able to sit up in the chair again, while very slowly some colour returns to his face.

'What happened, Willick?'

'My foot slipped under the peedie lawn tractor when the blades were turning,' he says as matter-of-factly as ever.

'Why didn't you phone me?'

'Never thought. I just jumped into the car and came here.'

Time and time again I've told folks not to do this, as neither of us might be here, but it still happens. I've always got the pager and the car radio so I can be contacted. I am just about to say this when Willick stands up to leave.

'Ah no, Willick, we'll just let you rest a while until I'm sure you've properly recovered. Come through to the kitchen and we'll get some tea made.'

'No. I'll just sit here,' he says and refuses to move.

Tea and scones seem to be doing the job, though. Either that or the period of unconsciousness has affected him. Willick chats away as he demolishes a second scone.

'We never thanked you for the cabbages after the dentist's visit.'

'Well, they're from the Laird's garden so never worry. Did I ever tell you the story of the rabbits?' He continues: 'Local folks would trap the rabbit for the pot until one time, so the story goes, the Laird decided all the rabbits were his, along with everything else. He forbid the folks to take the rabbits.' Willick's indignity shows as he says this. 'This wasn't so grand for the hill folks, who had no land and who relied on the wild rabbits for food. Anyway, nothing was said for a while until one moonless night a group of boys gathered on the shore carrying sacks. Each sack was carefully taken to the wall surrounding the Laird's garden and emptied quietly over it. Then everyone left.' Even before the next part of the tale, there's a delight which shows in his face. You could tell something good was going to happen. 'When the Laird took his usual morning stroll through the gardens next day they were bare, not a vegetable or flower to be seen. There was, however, a profusion of rabbits sleeping on the remaining grass. I suppose the boys thought they were being helpful bringing the Laird his rabbits and saving him looking for them on the hill.'

Even after all this time, I'm never sure if I'm being told the truth or just a story. It is a good story though.

'Right, Doc, I'll get away home now.'

'I'll take you back, Willick, you can't drive with that foot bandaged.'

'It'll be fine, don't you worry, I'll just use the other foot.'

Eventually we compromise, and he lets me put my bike into his Mini Metro while I drive him home.

The weather isn't so kind this autumn, with several periods of rain and gales blowing across the peat bog. Whether it is the damp or not we're not sure, but a few weeks after Willick cut his foot, Martin is in trouble with his asthma. It's not been bad since we took him off cow's milk but he's been up most of last night and isn't improving today; if anything, he's getting worse. Shifting the tray with its model of a tiny Vesuvius, it's time for another examination. I'm not sure why I decided we should make a model of Vesuvius out of plasticine and bicarbonate of soda but we did. The mountain frothed with white lava when the rain of vinegar hit it. Unfortunately, the little bedroom now smells like a chip shop.

Switching off the nebulizer, the little machine delivering the medication to open his airways, we pull up his pyjama top while I listen again to his chest.

'Take some big breaths again, pal, while I have a listen.'

Except big breaths aren't really happening. Short shallow breaths are. Not a great sign at this stage in treatment. After several hours of inhaled medication, supplemented by tablets of prednisolone designed to reduce the inflammation in the airways, Martin should be breathing a little more slowly now, more easily. He's not and I'm running out of things to give him.

'Okay, pal, just a few more breaths.'

'I'll ... try ... Dad.'

Listening to the middle of his lungs at the back, I can hear those three words clearly through the stethoscope. They should be muffled a little, like listening through a sponge. It is a sure sign he has pneumonia, the muck and rubbish of the infection blocking his airways, allowing the sounds to transmit clearly through the solid lung.

'Right, let's try something else, Mr Vesuvius builder. Pop these on your tongue and suck them until they're gone. We'll give the other stuff a bit more time to work, too.'

'OK ... Dad.' And, 'I ... need ... to ... pee.'

I carry him across the Heatherlea Badlands and Stairwell Rise to the toilet, sitting him on the loo and holding him up before carrying him back to bed. Briefly, he looks out of the window at his brothers playing football in the garden as sad envy registers in his eyes.

'I ... want ... to ...'

'Not yet, pal. In a little while maybe.'

Downstairs in the kitchen Maggie and I have a chat.

'How's he doing now?' she asks.

'Not much better, just the same really. I've given him some homeopathic treatment with his antibiotic but we may need to fly him out.'

'At least the weather is fine for the plane if we need to call it. Should he go now before it gets dark?'

'I'm not sure,' I say. 'I can't really think straight.'

'I'll sit with him, you take a break for a bit.'

'I'll go out and walk, I need to clear my head.'

A patient in Martin's position would usually be in hospital but technically there's not much more they will do for him. How confident am I to wait? How confident is he that I know what I'm doing? Not that he really has a choice, he simply has to trust me.

The walk down to Mill Bay isn't long and I'm soon on the beach, where I watched the Arctic tern flying freely, lazily, then stopping abruptly and focussing, before diving sharply on its prey. Carefully judging each movement before it acts. It will be on its way to the other side of the world now, still critically reading the seas below, watching for the tiny movements suggesting fish and eels moving beneath.

A gentle breeze rustles the grass on the shore, just a breath, not a hint of gales out to sea like before. The waves beat a steady, unhurried rhythm on the shore. There's no sign of tension down here. I let the breeze ruffle through my hair, feel its touch briefly on my cheek as I try to think.

'His pulse was down a little from an hour ago,' I hear myself say, 'a tiny movement in the right direction. His hands were warmer and his lips not so pale.'

Little movements, changes in direction, can they be trusted? It is difficult to be objective with your family but I have no choice either. Like Martin, I have to trust myself. If I phone another doctor, they won't take the risk, they'll just tell me to fly him in to hospital so they can actually see him. They won't trust what I tell them, they will want first-hand information. In their position I would want it, too. So I have to make the decisions. Walking back up the road to the house, I've made my choice. We'll wait another two hours and if there's no further improvement we fly.

Pushing open the door into the kitchen I stop dead. Martin is sitting in the armchair beside the stove, reading a book.

'Hi, Dad. I'm feeling better.'

'How? What did Mum do? What did she give you?'

'Nothing. Just juice.'

'Could the homeopathic medication have done that?' asks Maggie with a smile.

'In theory yes. That's why I chose it but I wasn't expecting it to work that quickly.'

'Can I go through and watch telly now please, Dad?'

'Yes. Sure, on you go. Stay wrapped up. No, wait, come here.'

Placing my stethoscope back on his chest, the area of pneumonia is still there but the air is flowing freely into the rest of his lungs so I let him go and play. I'm glad the signs of pneumonia haven't changed, proving my diagnosis wasn't wrong. Thank goodness I didn't make a call and arrange an ambulance flight. That would have been embarrassing, another neurotic doctor overanxious about his child and becoming out of touch, stuck out there on his island. Wrapped up in all the analysis of little changes in breathing, in pulse and colour, beneath all these things is something worse than clinical stupidity. Worse than overconfidence or medical machismo. It is the paralysing fear of embarrassment stopping us asking for help, making us delay calling for assistance.

Over the next week, Martin improves steadily but needs repeat doses of his homeopathic medication when his energy tails off. Gradually, his pneumonia clears over the next fortnight and he is right as rain again.

The longer nights have come round once more so again I've time to read. This year, I've ordered a series of seven books on outer space, entitled 'A Voyage through the Universe'. The nights are so clear and the sky so dark, every single star seems visible. I treated myself to a telescope for my birthday, just so I could look more closely at the night sky and already this autumn I've seen the four visible moons around Neptune. There is so much more to learn, so settling in front of the open peat fire – our own peat this year, cut from the bank behind the house – the first book lies open on my knee.

Halfway through the first chapter the phone rings. The voice on the other end is hysterical, high-pitched screaming alternating with sobbing. 'He has gone wild; he's got the poker; he's cut himself already; he's wild angry; you have to come!'

'Maggie, I'm going to have to go out, something is up with those folks staying at the hostel. He's cut himself already and is waving a poker, threatening to attack her.'

'Those ones doing the bird survey? They seemed okay when they were in to see me last week. She just needed more contraceptive pills.'

'I know. I'll go and see what's happened.'

'You should take someone with you; phone Magnus.'

'Maybe but that might make things worse, the police turning up. I'll go alone.'

'Call me and let me know you're okay.'

'I'll call in twenty minutes. If I don't, ask Magnus to come and find me.'

*

The youth hostel sits just over the hill, in a little valley, shielded from wind, rain and radio signals, making my car radio useless if I need help. I let the car coast quietly to a halt, killing the lights long before arriving. Stepping silently from the car, I stop and listen. I want to be sure of what is happening before I dive in. The moonless blackness of the night lies thickly around the wooden hostel; there's nothing to see. So I listen. The shore birds are silent as they listen, too. Listen to the swearing and shouting and crashing of furniture from inside the wooden hut. Maybe I should have brought Magnus with me.

In the hallway of the hut, the phone is still hanging off the hook where the woman left it after calling me. Carefully, I replace the receiver I might need quickly later and let myself quietly into the sitting room, where the focus of the uproar is coming from. The man is pacing wildly around, waving the poker taken from the stove in the middle of the room. A torrent of vitriol is pouring from him while blood slowly drips from his other hand. Presumably, it was cut on the smashed table lamp lying on the floor, still stupidly shining yellow light up into his contorted face. The woman is still screaming at him from the shadows on the other side of the room. Both are clearly the worse for drink.

'Aye, aye. There's a hell of a noise in here,' I say, as I slowly move in from the doorway, all the time looking directly at him.

My unexpected appearance has wrong-footed both of them, as the torrent ceases. They hadn't considered a third player, so quickly, in their orgy of abuse. The man pauses briefly, taking time to suck air through his pursed lips before trying to recruit me into the fight with another torrent of abuse aimed at the woman. Careering round the table between us, he faces up to me, breathing whisky into my face while still brandishing the hot poker. I've no intention of playing this game.

'Aye, there's definitely too much noise,' I say, and still never letting my gaze fall from his face I slowly sit down on the dining chair I've moved just a bit nearer the open door.

The whites of his eyes are suffused with red, the tiny blood vessels pulsating with his rapid heartbeat. They don't matter – it's his pupils I must watch. If they dilate, grow larger with the excitement and adrenalin, then I will move quickly to the door. He narrows his eyes, a puzzled look unlocking the contortions of anger as he considers me sitting in the middle of his battlefield. Slowly his pupils constrict, just a little, the adrenalin subsiding a fraction. Hours of watching patients' faces when I've had them in a hypnotic trance pay off. The minuscule movements of facial muscles are the telltale signs of stress or relaxation. It's time for the next move.

'Somebody go and put the kettle on.'

The sheer incongruity of me sitting down in the middle of this violence, asking for a cup of tea, finally breaks the spell. He breaks down in tears in front of me, overwhelmed by emotion and, shaking uncontrollably, he sinks into the chair beside me. The woman, thinking she sees her chance to take control and have the last word, draws a breath to start the battle again.

'We'll have that tea now!' my voice emphatic and uncompromising. 'Right, now, let's take that poker away, eh! Show me your hand and we'll sort out some stitches, I think.'

I'm reluctant to leave the room and call Maggie but I must or else Magnus will arrive and things may get tricky again. Lifting the receiver while standing in the doorway, I dial home.

'Just me. Things are fine.'

'You're late. I nearly called Magnus.'

'Sorry. Things took a bit longer to settle down than I thought.'

'I knew they would.'

After I've cleaned and stitched the man's hand, we agree to meet tomorrow at the surgery and talk through tonight's events. I doubt if I'll see either of them again, though. They have one more day of the bird survey to complete then they leave the island. They'll have to. The island is exposing the problems between them, the wind scarifying the sands, peeling back the layers and revealing the bedrock of resentment and anger that lies below.

18

Understanding

They say when you toss a coin in the air your mind is made up while the coin still spins. You know what side you want to be 'up' before it lands. While that is probably true, it leaves the process only half-done. The other side of the coin, the decision, the act, the situation you avoided will still need to be dealt with at some point. Life is never one-sided. The exact opposite to what you hoped for is literally only a flip of the coin away. It's no use planning in straight lines, connecting single events, looking only at the one side of the coin. In this remote landscape the constant wind, life itself, will toss your plans into the sea.

Was I lucky when I tried to control the flames of emotion at the hostel last night? As it turns out, I read the bursts of sound, flickers of movement and gestures correctly. It was dangerous for a while, though, with that coin spinning in the air before it landed as I'd hoped. The weapon laid aside, anger subsiding a little as the frenzy of the moment gave way to despair. Like any fire, the inferno takes a little while to die down completely, threatening to reignite with the least fanning of the embers. His wife was keen to fan the flames again once she had me as an ally, or so she thought.

There's an exhilaration in the unknown, in allowing things to develop as they will. Enjoying that excitement can be dangerous, making you overconfident and preventing you seeing what's really happening. I suppose that's why I sit down in the middle of these events if I can. Taking myself to a different place, literally lowering my viewpoint, giving myself a little space to think and assess. Many times it takes me nearer my patient, bringing them down to me and stopping their pacing in agitation. We can meet as equals when we sit together.

Thrill-seeking isn't a good way for a doctor to work. I'm aware I might not be able to read events in future as well as I did the last time. This thought lingers in my mind as I step out of the car at the top of the little hill above the surgery. I've come up here to check the car radio link with the hospital, something that should be done each week but I don't always remember. Today the checks can wait a little longer; the view is spectacular.

Looking south over our island neighbours, it seems as though the sea has disappeared, drawn back from the land, so all that's in view are brown and purple hills woven into each other like a rumpled patchwork quilt. Each island is connected as far as the eye can see. Thin mist softens the edges, as the hills roll into the hazy distance, as if you can walk to the furthest horizon and never feel a wave splash over your feet. I let the landscape surround me, allowing myself to sink down into the comfort of the quilt, bridging moments in my life. I've been here before, in this landscape, it's where I was brought up, in the fields and hills of the Borders of Scotland, far from the sea. In this landscape I am what I dreamed about being when I was aged nine: a country GP with my own practice. A GP confident enough to calm the fears of a father whose son is having an asthma attack not responding to treatment. My son. My dream didn't include working in such a wild and beautiful place as this.

'Balfour Hospital, Balfour Hospital, this is Eday one. Testing. Testing.'

Crackle, hiss, hiss ... silence

'Balfour Hospital, Balfour Hospital, this is Eday one. Testing. Testing.'

Crackle, hiss, crackle ... silence.

The signal from my car radio drifts out into the ether, never to return. Some days are like this but I have to try, part of making sure that if the tossed coin lands 'wrong side up' I have the ability to call for help in this remote place. If the phones go down, this radio is my only communication with the outside world.

'Dosh the sound'sh blow away in the wind, Daddy?'

'Oh, sorry, Peedie, I forgot you were there. No, they can't do that but some days the signal bounces away into the sky.'

'Just like my hor'sh when it's arsing ...'

'Peedie!'

'... being bad?'

'Yes, a bit like that. On days when the weather is nice the signals run away. Right, you try to see if it will work.'

There's a huge grin on his face as he says ...

'Balfour Ho'shpital, Balfour Ho'shpital ... what's next?'

'This is Eday one. Testing. Testing.'

'Th'ish is Eday one. Teshing. Teshing.'

Hiss, crackle ...

'Ed ... ne, this's Balfour Hos ... receiving y ... loud and clear.'

Peedie's eyes shine and he claps his hands.

'Thank you, Balfour Hospital. Eday one, over and out!'

Turning the car on the rough ground at the top of the track, the stones crunching and sparking under each tyre, Peedie is firmly wedged between my legs to let him steer us down the hillside. All the boys have loved doing this, holding grimly on to the steering wheel, refusing to let it go and inevitably failing to navigate the twists and bends of the stony trail. Time and time again we reverse back from the edge of a ditch as I wrestle the car straight and off we go again. Down by the roadside again, Peedie scrambles into the back and straps himself into his booster seat.

'That was great, Daddy, better than riding my hor'sh!'

I suppose they all grow up, don't they? Looks like Peedie's wheelie horse may be going out to pasture soon. Dropping Peedie off at the house, I continue north to visit Ken, who has been bedridden with sciatica for four days.

Ken and Sue moved years ago, in one of the early waves of migration from the south, to the only land they could readily afford. Fertile pasture on mainland Orkney is and always has been at a premium compared with North Isles settlements. It's not easy for outsiders to gain a foothold on good land. Orcadians move in from the isles to the mainland, leaving poorer land open for new prospectors and there was good reason for Ken and Sue's land being available. Nestling in the curve of Calf Sound, the land is trapped, held fast between the peat bog of Bomo to the south and the steep rocky shore of the sound. The ground looks as it behaves – irascible. A damp, grumbling mixture of thin soil and rock, covered by coarse pasture. Never truly green, even in summer, the pasture is flecked with grey and brown all year. Patches of bog cotton blown from around Mill Loch in the southerly gales mingle with 'soft rush', a spiky reed, and tough scrubby grass. Even the name of the rushes is derisive, 'soft rush' being a coarse, reed-like, indestructible grass. No wonder old maps give the crofts at the north end names such as 'Purgatory', 'Gravesend' and 'Furrowend'.

In this no man's land of farming they work a croft, with cows in the byre, sheep on the rough grazing, a pig in a sty two miles away, more sheep on the West Side Road. Nothing is easy in this setting; any success is fought for with determination and hard graft. The least let-up in the work and the land fights back.

Swinging the little car on to the farm track, I can see the row of guard-ducks lined up along the roof of the croft house – comical-looking Muscovy ducks, with red lumpy faces and badly painted black and white bodies. As if they had been made in a beginner's pottery class, prodded and squashed into a rough duck shape then spattered with paint. They watch me with feigned disinterest as I climb out of the car.

Sue is straining fresh goat's milk into a bright clean steel pail as I let myself into the kitchen.

'Hi Sue, how's he doing today?'

She half-smiles a reply. Ken is not the best patient.

'Just the same. He can't move but he's going round the west side once you've been. He needs to feed the sheep.'

'Really, that should help a lot with his pain. Let me see what I can do. He's through in the room as usual?'

'Same place. I'll sort the milk while you see him.'

'Ta.'

We've been buying milk from Sue to supplement our own supply. I'm not quite good enough yet at milking our own goats to keep us all going.

'Aye Ken, how are you doing today? Sue says you're going round the west side later.'

'Your medicine's no bloody use, I can't move hardly.'

A point he reinforces by trying to rise up from the bed they've dragged into the living room.

'Aaaah, bloody hell, sorry, Doc!'

'Right, right, stay still just now while I take a look at you. How are you managing to go to the loo? Everything working fine?'

'Once I'm bloody upright it's fine.'

'Ken!' Sue has finished with the milk. 'Ken, mind your language.'

'Sorry, Doc, it's just so bloody sore as soon as I move. Right down the back of this leg.'

Bizarrely, he appears to be wearing a boiler suit in bed, a clear sign that he has not been lying resting as I told him to. Once I've carefully removed the strange bed attire, I take a good look at him. He is as thin and wiry as the land he works, almost as incorrigible too. The spasm of pain I cause by gently lifting his right leg courses down to his fingertips, and he screws the bed sheet into a ball.

'That feels fine, Doc, just give me jab and I'll get those sheep fed.'

'I can see that, Ken, you can let the bed sheet go now,' I say, looking across at Sue. 'There's no bloody way you're going anywhere today. I've told you before, this will only fix with rest. It's either that or I put you into hospital. Which do you want?'

Sometimes incorrigible needs to meet its match.

'Okay, right, fine, Doc. But what about the sheep? Sue can't shift the bales to the bottom of the field.'

'I'll do it, if it will make you stay in bed.'

'You can't do that. I'll ask Billy if he can.'

'Don't be daft, I'm here anyway, I'll sling the bales in the boot. Now shut up and turn away from me while I give you this jab.'

There's a technique called 'mirroring' which I learned about, where you match the speech patterns and body movements of your patient as you respond. Apparently, we all do it if we're in tune with another person. I seem to do it naturally. It definitely makes a difference in getting a point across.

'Okay, Ken, that should ease things back a bit for you now. Let's be clear, though, when I come by tomorrow I want to see you wearing clothes and not a boiler suit. I'll away and get that hay now, get those sheep fed before the storm comes in again. It'll be rough again tonight.'

'Thanks, Doc, sorry about my bloody language.' There's a glint in his eye as he says it. 'Put the bale in the little shed at the bottom of the field – keeps it drier there for them.'

'Will do.'

'Oh, and mind the gate at the top of the field, it's just thick mud there, it'd take your Wellies right off.'

'I'll be fine. Right, Sue, show me the hay and we'll chuck it in the boot.'

Around the back of the house Sue and I put two bales into the boot of the car. Watching her move, I'm struck by how she looks much older than her years. She's strong, lifting and swinging the bales into the boot, but her back is painful too. She struggles to carry the bale over the yard but won't let me help. Incorrigible and determined are well matched. It's her hands that really tell the story though. Once almost elegant fingers are now thickened, patches of callus marking where the rough plastic binder twine has eaten into her skin. Somehow it appears different from Ivan, whose hands were equally used to hard work. Digging holes for fencing, clearing ditches, working with the soil. His hands seemed to match the land, reflect its nature. Sue's hands are scarred by the work, as if fighting against something. I wonder whose dream it was to move to this harsh north end croft.

Driving back down through the island, I'm struck once again by the fragility of life. By the speed with which the course of its path can change. A tiny, probably only 2mm fragment of the pressure cushion in Ken's spine, his vertebral disc, has ruptured to press on to a nerve, completely disabling him. Making him and all those around him vulnerable. Sheep that depend on him for feed, cows in the sheds, chickens and ducks. All in jeopardy from a tiny 2mm protrusion in his spine. If he was single, as many of the men are, he would be in real trouble. It's quite clear that, without any fuss, the women are the glue in this place. Spanning kitchen and byre, children and cattle, the unseen strength holding everything together. Is it women who truly understand the nature of this island? An island holding back the North Sea and cradling its own calf across the sound, sheltering it. No, I don't think so: they're just a different expression of the same battle for survival in an unforgiving place.

Back at the house, there's time for a cup of tea before changing into my boiler suit and heading out with the bales. The sheep are on the West Side Road, about two miles from Heatherlea, in a steep field that slides down to the shore. The rain has started already, the rising wind battering sheets of water against the windscreen, defying the wipers to cope. Pulling the car up at the roadside, being careful to stay on the stony road margin, I shelter briefly behind the door before stepping out into the wind. Carefully clambering through the gate, staying out of the mud which is deep enough to drown a sheep, I start to trudge down the field with a full bale of hay to the little feeding hut at the bottom, escorted by grey, sodden sheep who hirple with a foot-rotted limp behind me. My boiler suit is soaked through, covered in thick, sticky mud as the wind cuts my face with slaps of seaweed, blown from the equally sodden grey seashore. A sharp, knifing stab in my back makes me wince as I lift the bale over the threshold of the shed. There's no way Ken would have made it here. Or would he?

The shed is damp inside too, and as I slice through the orange binder twine to break open the bale, the wind whistles through the holes in the roof while rain soaks the floor beside the shattered window. The stale ammoniacal smell of wet sheep persists despite the wind, as I look around in the half-light for a clean place to lay the bale down. There isn't one. There's a constant piping sound too, insistent and irritating, out of time with the gale. Tracking the sound to my pocket, my heart misses several beats. My pager is going off. My pager never goes off; why would Maggie page me? What has happened that she can't cope with? Why am I in the middle of a bloody field when it goes off? Nothing ever happens here that needs me paged!

The climb back to the car is screamingly painful as the wind literally refuses to let me breathe, sucking air away from me, pushing me down time and again into the mud and slime of the grey-green matted hillside. I try to run but it's not possible. What has happened? No one ever pages me!

'Balfour Hospital, Balfour Hospital, this is Eday one. Over!'

'Balfour Hospital, Balfour Hospital, this is Eday one. Over!'

I can't even hear the hiss and crackle over the wind noise.

'Balfour Hospital, Balfour Hospital, this is Eday one. OVER!'

I'm on the wrong side of the bloody hill! I floor the little engine in the VW Polo and tear round the West Side Road, not caring about oncoming traffic. There won't be any on a night like this.

'Eday one, Eday one, this is Balfour Hospital. Over!'

'Eday one, you paged me, over!' I reply, while simultaneously taking the junction between the West Side Road and the main road with one hand on the wheel.

'No sorry, Eday one, I've not paged you. Will I call your house?'

'No thanks, I'm nearly back now. Eday one, out!'

Abandoning the car at the gate and seeing no light on in the surgery, I tear into the kitchen and see Maggie ... standing calmly at the stove, cooking tea. Megan is sleeping peacefully in her bouncer as Matthew gently rocks her. The dog comes up, wagging his tail. They all look round, surprised, as I stand covered in mud on the doormat.

'What's happened?' Maggie asks anxiously.

'You paged me, I was at the bottom of the field and my pager went off!' I say, taking the pager from my pocket as I tell her. I look at the pager and notice the little red light is still flashing ... the little red light that tells you the battery is about to die! The light that comes with a slower bleep ... bleep ... bleep to tell you to replace the battery!

'I'm going for a shower!'

I should have known nothing ever really happens that would need two of us urgently.

*

The wild north-easterly winds bring the edge of winter with them now. There's a feeling of newness, of something changing as the weeks drift by. The wind suggests a change of viewpoint, that we should look at things a different way. The same wind that shook and buffeted the little plane while it tried to prevent Maggie leaving to go to Aberdeen now brings new things for us to see. In the tiny trees which hide from the wind behind the stone dykes in the garden there's an occasional blink of orange. I can see it as I look out of the sitting-room window. There it is again, only a brief but deliberate wink of colour against the browns and greens of the remaining autumn leaves.

Saturday morning breakfast of home-made bread and fresh eggs from our ducks descends into chaos as the tribe charge through to the sitting room.

'Can you see, right at the bottom of the garden, almost against the wall.'

'I saw it, just then, an orange flash. It's eyes, something with eyes in the tree!' Matthew is always quick to spot things.

'T'sh it a snake?' asks Peedie, with his eyes nearly as big as the thing in the tree.

'Look really closely, tell me what else you see. What shape is it? What colour?'

'It's a bird, a huge brown bird. You can hardly see it at all,' says Martin. 'Is it an owl, Dad?'

'Exactly, but the question is, which kind of owl? Look again, take your time, it will tell you its name.'

'It'sh a snake owl!'

'No, not quite, keep looking carefully.'

'It's a tufted owl, it's got tufts on its head. Is that its ears?' asks Mike, describing with precision what he sees. Mike is always precise.

'Absolutely correct. It's called a long-eared owl but the ears are actually just tufts of feathers to make it look fierce. We'll stay out of the garden today and let it rest. It's travelling to its wintering ground, I think. Perhaps far across the North Sea. We're just a stopping-off point. We'll leave it in peace. Let's go for a walk round Mill Loch instead and see what else we see.'

It has taken a while for me to allow myself to wander very far from the house. The radio in the car remains useless most of the time, despite me fitting a bigger aerial. The sense of responsibility for all the folks on the island held me back, especially now I know them personally. People still insist on turning up unannounced at the house, like Willick when he was bleeding severely from his cut foot. Gradually, though, I'm settling to the different rhythm, the slower pace of life here, and we can walk further from home as a family now.

Today is a glorious, blue-sky day as our bundle of children in duffel coats and hats wander round Mill Loch and over the hill. Martin tears past on his bike, followed by a wobbly Mike, who's just learned enough in the goat paddock to try it out on the road. It's quiet now, as we walk along the north shore of the loch. The loons have all headed out to sea for the winter, taking their mourning cry with them. As we pass the spot on the hill where Ivan died, I stand still for a minute. Maggie knows why. Patients sometimes think they are just one among many but they aren't. Each life stays with us. I still remember the first patient I was with when she died. A tiny scrap of a lady on my first medical ward who had no one to be with her. She was simply dying of old age and beginning the sleep that she needed. The student nurse was too nervous, uncertain what to do, and quickly rushed away to some important task. I just sat for the little while it took for the lady to pass away. Nothing complex, just sitting down beside her, being with her while she slept away. Final breaths are unnerving at first, so much like gasps that you feel the person is waking up again. I still wish I could have been with Ivan too, at the end.

Over the top of the hill there's a field that is full of the biggest mushrooms we have seen. Soon Megan's pushchair is crammed with the giant brown dinner plates that Maggie will turn into an almost purple soup. The boys refused to eat it the first time we picked them, the colour was so lurid. I suppose we're all too used to the sanitized tins of Campbell's Cream of Mushroom to really understand what fresh food should be like.

Ahead of us on the road, for several hundred yards now, a blackbird has been hopping along. Always flying a little further in front as we get near. Looking closer, I see it has a faint white collar on the front of its neck. A ring ouzel. Another of the birds brought in on the north-easterly wind, resting before continuing its journey south for the winter. This bird won't fly as far as my Arctic tern; the ouzel will stop and bask in winter sun in the mountains of Tunisia.

There is a sense of everything leaving the island just now. Not a disturbing feeling, more a feeling of relaxation from the activities of summer. An exhalation. Visitors in the hostel have gone and the boats serving our little island are back to the winter timetable now. One cargo boat a week will come on Wednesdays, depending on the weather. The birds are all moving off too, seeking less harsh places to winter. Leaving us, the islanders, to look after the place until they return. Only the seals will stay with us, hauling up on the Holms to breed, their haunting calls drifting across the sea.

My daydream is broken sharply as the ouzel flies off, frightened by Martin whizzing past on his bike, followed at a short distance by a precarious but determined Mike.

'Mike, stop now. Before the hill goes down!' I shout uselessly into the wind.

Martin's head disappears round the bend and sinks down the hill as I run after Mike to try to catch him. Too late, gravity has taken effect and Mike is accelerating, against his will, down towards the sea.

'Martin! Try to stop Mike before ...' Ah, it's all right, Martin has seen what's happening. 'Martin! No, not like that.'

Realizing that Mike is in danger of hurtling down the hill and crashing horribly, Martin has jumped off his bike and placed it sideways across the path of his careering brother. The effect is instantaneous, catastrophic and graceful at the same time. Ramming into the makeshift crash barrier, Mike has his downward trajectory converted into an upward one, as he performs a beautiful arched somersault into the nearby ditch. Breathlessly, I catch up with them.

'Are you all right? Are you hurt?'

Lying upside down in the ditch, his cycle helmet at a jaunty angle over one eye, a smile broadens across his face.

'I have stopped now,' he says.

Mike is always precise.

After another uneventful week of routine – cleaning the little pharmacy, checking the orders, organizing the delivery of the annual flu jabs which Trevor, my locum, will give when he comes in October, there's a little time to tidy the yard and admire the world's smallest peat stack.

Peats that have been carefully dried and barrowed back from the hill in July are now sitting in a circular stack beside the animal hospital shed. Carefully covered with turf, cut to make a waterproof roof for the winter, they are a thing of pride and amusement. I see the smiles passing over the faces of the locals as they walk past my efforts at island living. Erland just nodded when he saw it as he passed on his tractor, loaded with peat ready to be tidied and stacked with precision once more. I won't care what they all think when I'm sitting beside the fire this winter, reading the next series of books I've ordered.

The nicotiana plants I bought at Jenny's sale of work in August have flowered beautifully and even attracted a hummingbird on several of the late September evenings, or so we thought at first. All we could see was a small bird-like creature, smaller than a wren, flitting between the blooms, hovering with rapidly beating wings while dipping a long, fine beak into the nectar ponds at their base. It was the strangest thing. Researching the books on the bookshelf and asking a few of the folks in the surgery, it turned out the bird is actually a moth. A hummingbird hawkmoth that is addicted to the scent of nicotiana plants. A tobacco addict. These fascinating moths are rarely seen this far north and seeing one is said to be a good omen. We've seen it lots of times.

Just as I reach down to pull the remains of the plant up and put it in the compost, someone leans over the surgery gate. Then opening the gate slightly, they say, 'I don't feel too great, Doc,' before sliding slowly on to the concrete path.

I didn't hear them arrive, they were almost silent. Too silent. All true emergencies arrive quietly. A quietness surrounding serious illness that is unnerving, similar to the calm before a storm, where the imperceptible change in the lap of waves on the shore and a shiver in the windblown grass signals trouble ahead. Noise is traumatic, painful and alive. Silence is deadly. In this microsecond of silence, my heart rate rises.

Words can't capture the remoteness, the sheer isolation I feel deep inside in that moment when the world decides to miss a beat. Here on the island, at the birth of death, there is only you, alone and with no second chance to change the course of events. Maggie will help, of course, but the responsibility is mine. In other places you can look away if you choose, refusing to play your part. The crash team will come; the ambulance will arrive; you can just assist. The island has no such luxury, no soft centre to nestle in while you watch and wait. The harsh, unforgiving reality of the rolling hills and shore-caressing sea is crueller than any cityscape, with its opportunities for multiple excuses.

In the instant the day shudders at the unfolding emergency, there is fear. Deep in the bedrock that formed me, at my very core, there is fear. The kick of fear doctors never talk about to each other because no one has given us the language to use. The fear that is never taboo because for it to be so we would have to acknowledge it existed. This is not unstructured panic, useless and self-defeating – that has no place in what I do. The inquietude is liquid, molten, burning so far down inside me that at times I'm not sure I recognize it is there. But it is. From when I was a young boy, the fear and fascination of medicine mesmerized me, captivating me, until the day I said, 'I want to be a doctor because I like helping people.' Each time I learned a new technique, a skill, I let the fascination bury the fear, until at last I no longer felt it. Until the day the earth shakes once more.

The heat from the molten disquiet, the fear of failure, spawns everything I know, bringing it to life and available to use. The methodical calm of the family GP; tiny movements and sounds captured in hypnotic detail; books on the shelves of my memory; simulation and practice; the smell of formaldehyde in anatomy class; sky and cloud patterns; the wind. All these cascade into 'now' as the moment of fear, the microsecond of silence breaks into thousands and I know what to do.

As Maggie and I work, the rhythm of our activities takes over. The practised familiar routine played out every day by doctors everywhere. Doing helps. Our capability is as good as it can be. With the addition of the ECG machine we can monitor and treat most eventualities for the short while we wait on the plane. We manage the pain with intravenous morphine, provide oxygen with a high-flow mask; thin the blood a little with aspirin; blood pressure is controlled; urine output is measured. Alertness makes the fear redundant, anticipation is key now. Slow methodical calm as emergency drugs are set out in rows ready for use. Simulations run mentally in real time – if this, then that. Patterns recognized and prepared for, as there will be no time to search for an injection if the need arises. The pattern isn't clear, though. There is a problem with blood supply to the heart, at least that's what the ECG is telling me. But! Sometimes that's as far as I get – But! It niggles in my mind, that word, like a sentry on duty looking out for the unexpected.

Then I watch and wait. The harsh reality that everything that can be done, has been done. Anticipation is complete. The air ambulance has been ordered, the hospital spoken to, the transfer party assembled. Others wait outside, ready to move us to the airstrip. Maggie has gone to check on Megan and the boys. Claire is smoking, outside in the yard. During all the frenetic activity, I've been able to communicate with my patient through quick looks, fleeting touches, and brief words of reassurance. Tiny movements of their hands and eyes have signalled their questions, as exhaustion prevents anything more. In this hiatus before the transfer to Kirkwall, when we could take the time to talk more, we find there is nothing say. The two of us caught in this moment together, alone with our fear.

Rhythm – the beat continues: re-examine; recheck;

reassess. Pulse; blood pressure; capillary refill; pain level. I carefully check and recheck in a surgery that seems full now, although there are only two of us here. The torn examination couch, once dust-covered and tired, is surrounded by oxygen cylinders, drip stands and the ECG machine. The desk is hidden under a paper sheet and carefully laid out with vials and syringes. The centrifuge in the pharmacy spins the baseline bloods to send with my patient. I can't do anything with the samples but they'll help later as comparators. All of this activity takes place under the watchful eye of the wall clock, precisely recording the passing time.

Is this a heart attack? Keep looking. Something has changed. A new sign brought to the surface and exposed. With this new sign comes a memory, the page of a half-remembered book that I cannot read clearly. A brief paragraph touching on the unusual and stirring disquiet again. There is sadness in this emergent blemish, an inevitability in the half-remembered words. For now, I discard the mark as it changes nothing in the treatment and sit down beside my patient, listening to the steady beep ... beep ... beep of the machine while we watch and wait once more.

Slowly, above the quiet rumble of conversation surrounding the small group of people gathered outside, the hum of a bee carries across on the wind. Gradually, the buzz grows into the distant sound of an aircraft engine.

Making sure we know he's here, Dave roars the plane over the surgery and down the hill to the airstrip.

Gravel crunches under our feet as we carry the stretcher over to the plane. There is nothing simple or slick about putting a stretcher into the aircraft, which was never designed to become an ambulance. Most of the seats have been removed, with only two left for the ambulanceman and me, leaving no space for passengers. The stretcher poles are manhandled over and around the remaining seats, then fixed into position and secured for the flight. Carefully arranging the drips and monitor, I hesitate for a moment. Although I've known from the beginning what I will do, there's a final moment of uncertainty. A balancing of risk before I allow the doors of the plane to close behind me.

The wind shakes the brittle winter grasses as I walk away from the plane. Standing beside the car, I watch the plane turn to face the inevitability in the north wind before it rises into the sky without me. My seat taken by another. This is a journey two people need to take together.

'Balfour Hospital, Balfour Hospital, this is Eday one. Over.'

'Balfour Hospital. Go ahead, Eday one.'

'Eday one. That's the flight just leaving the airstrip. Is the receiving doctor in the hospital now?'

'Balfour Hospital. Yes, he's here.'

'Eday one. Thank you. I'll call him from my surgery. Eday one, out.'

Epilogue

The Sound of the Merry Dancers

As Christmas approaches, once more I pop in to see Jenny and discuss church services. Returning from making the obligatory cup of tea, she arranges herself on the two-seater settee, carefully plumping two brocade cushions before putting them to one side. So that's what happened to them after the August sale. I knew they wouldn't be wasted.

The reason for my visit is to ask if we could have a watchnight service this year on Christmas Eve. With Jenny's approval, I've managed to sort out the preaching properly now and have a free hand. She was in favour of the service and even offered to organize hot mince pies and tea afterwards. I wasn't sure how this was possible in a building with only gas lighting and no running water. It was then that the Orcadian twinkle came into Jenny's eye and you could see her think, *Boy, you just don't know anything, do you?*

'Ah, well,' she says, 'we'll see what can be done.'

I was about to ask more questions but we noticed the steamer coming down the sound again so it was time to go.

Christmas Eve and the church doesn't look so lonely tonight, as we walk up the grassy path to the front door. There are lots of cars parked outside and families from all over the island are slowly making their way up the hillside. Once inside the church, I leave the children with Maggie. A row of white-haired infants blending into brown-haired primary kids, all identically dressed in cream Arran knit cardigans sent by Aunty Betty to keep them warm in winter.

The atmosphere in the sanctuary has a magical feel to it, accentuated by the pale golden glow from the gas lamps. The mantles sing lightly above us, giving off the smell of childhood again, while the warming wax on the pews suggests bees and honey. The gentle rise and fall of hushed voices adds to the feeling of specialness, faces turning to each other and chatting, half-lit in the warm glow of the singing lamps.

Jenny says we're ready to start but I'm extremely worried now, as I turn and look towards the front of the church. I can just see Tommy's head above the old pedal organ and there's very definitely a column of smoke rising beside him. As I rush forwards everything becomes clear and I understand the twinkle in Jenny's eye when I asked about tea and mince pies after the service. Alongside Tommy, the glossy grey painted paraffin heater, carefully placed to ensure he doesn't freeze, is also warming a large steel kettle. Streams of warm steam flow from its spout and drift up in the gas light.

The service is a joy to take, although it's as well I chose not to go into the pulpit tonight. Baby Megan is refusing to do anything but cry unless I hold her in my arms. Slowly, the weight on my arm increases as she drifts off to sleep. I suppose it's all right to have a sleeping baby at the centre of a Christmas Eve service.

After the service finishes, a triumphant Jenny with ladies from the Guild serve hot drinks from the steaming kettles and warm home-made mince pies from trays wrapped in tin foil. All have been kept hot on the strategically placed paraffin stoves and there's enough for all fifty folk who have come to the service. The church is filled with the chatter of voices as folks munch their way through the festive food then say 'Merry Christmas' to each other, before heading back to peat fires and Christmas trees. Another thread of island history is woven into place.

As everyone melts into the night, the sky behind the little church clears of cloud. A deep velvet blackness falls all around me, touching the sea. Blackness broken not by starlight but clothed in ribbons of luminous green and yellow light streaming across the horizon. Tonight, the birds and their night-time shore songs are silent as the effervescent air comes alive with the shimmering tingle of sound.

Many people have seen the Merry Dancers – the Northern Lights – some not knowing what they are. Few, very few, have heard the electric beat of the solar winds. The sound of the Merry Dancers.

Beneath Electric Skies

I am Eid-ey,
The isthmus isle, the connector of tidal lands.

Through time I journey in the fierce northern seas.
I am
Flawed yet whole.
I live,
Drawing all to me, gathering them on my shores.
Holding them,
Testing them in the northern winds
until only the sea and the rich black peat remain.

The birds
Sing my shore songs
and the
Lips of the wind whisper
in my grass.

Yet few can hear the truth that lies
Beneath my electric skies.

Acknowledgements

I hope you read this part of the book because without the people below there wouldn't have been one! Everyone is part of this story, a story I could never have written without them.

So thank you to:

Laura Macdougall at United Agents – For having the trust and insight to realize that in all my ramblings there may just be a story to tell. Knowing almost nothing about me other than the fact that I go fishing, she allowed me to write badly, guiding me carefully until I stopped. Then I surprised myself by writing a book.

Nicki Crossley at Michael O'Mara Books – For taking the risk that my book was worth publishing and being gently ruthless with my words until it was. I am grateful to her for not only sorting out the words but also for crafting the whole book. Never judge a book by its cover but no one picks up a cover-less book – or a poorly set out, printed and marketed one.

Gabriella Nemeth has saved me from the pitfalls present in a debut manuscript with her excellent editing, indeed the whole MOM team have been great to work with. Just enough of a nudge to make things better but not too much to crowd me out. Doctors don't like crowds.

To all my family for letting me write about them as I saw them. Allowing me to overdramatize just a little for effect – but not much. Mostly to my wife and partner, Maggie, who has worked beside me since we first met in a surgical ward. Then she told me off for not doing my job properly and with a raise of an eyebrow she still does. She has another story to tell of our time on Eday, perhaps more powerful than mine – maybe one day we'll record that, too. Meanwhile, we'll just celebrate our thirty-eight years together and continue to write our own tale.

The people of Eday will never know how much they changed me, allowing me to understand what really matters in life. Unfortunately, almost all the people hidden in this book have passed on, so I can never thank them. This book is my way of saying thank you to them for showing me the only important thing in life is how we treat each other. This is what our survival, our happiness, depends on and nothing more.